Wellness on Time
Magazine

Issue 6

The
Ageing
Well
Edition

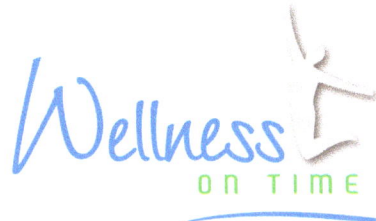

Wellness
ON TIME

wellnessontime.net

Wellness on Time
Magazine

Issue 6

Wellness on Time CEO, Founder, Publisher, Editor-in-Chief Natalie Pickett

Design Firestar Studios

Image credits Shutterstock, interview features supplied their own images, the archival photo of Thelma and Louise in Egypt on page 23 was supplied by the author, and the wise old owl image on page 24 is by Agto Nugroho on Unsplash.

Subscription, circulation and advertising enquiries info@wellnessontime.com

Advertising Partners

The Mineral Spa, Mineral Springs Hotel, Hepburn Springs, Australia page 9

The Indigenous Art Book page 14 • **Healing Haven** page 15

For information about becoming one of our Advertising Partners, email info@wellnessontime.com

Wellness on Time Magazine, Issue 6. ISBN: 978-0-6458943-5-6 published October 2024 by Wellness on Time, PO Box 738, Elsternwick VIC 3185 Australia. +61 412 568 215. ACN 168 942 238

© Wellness on Time MMXXIV www.wellnessontime.com

From the Editor

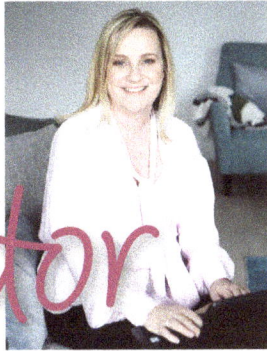

It's a pleasure to introduce you to our sixth edition of the *Wellness on Time Magazine* – the Ageing Well Edition.

The older I get, the more I've come to understand that one of the keys to achieving more is by doing less. I take time out to savour life's special moments, and I say 'No' to things that drain my energy, and an unconditional 'Yes!' to things that bring me joy. When we feel well in ourselves, we feel youthful. Our bodies are a miracle in design, but we are often not using them to their greatest potential. Less is more here too, because when we are moving in a way that creates ease of movement, the body is in harmony and things seem effortless.

One of my 'go to' modalities is Feldenkrais (aka Awareness Through Movement). This modality is about gentle movement that changes our habitual patterns to open new neural pathways that allow our bodies to move the way they are designed to. One of my biggest takeaways from this is that we often make things harder than they need to be. When I'm working on anything now and it seems hard, I ask myself, 'How can I make this easier?' Listening to how you feel is important. Taking steps each day to connect mind, body, and spirit helps bring us back into balance and restore a feeling of wellness.

I created 'Wellness on Time' in April 2014, and this year we're celebrating our 10 Year Anniversary! 'Make it easy, make it fun' is one of our mottos. After discovering ways to improve well-being, I wanted to show others how to easily integrate wellness activities into their lives too. That was the impetus to start Wellness on Time.

Wellness on Time is about connecting people to quality programs and products, to assist them to easily integrate wellness into their lives. We've had such a wonderful response since we added magazines and book publishing as the natural extension to the online wellness concept. I'm delighted and honoured to be publishing what we have included in this issue, and I am grateful to everyone who has shared their wisdom.

I'm a serial entrepreneur of 30 years and an international best-selling author. All of my businesses and my writing come from my passions and wanting to share knowledge with others. This is a global magazine with a global audience. We have writers from all over the world sharing their valuable knowledge, insights and stories about what they do, where to find support, and suggestions of ways to improve well-being.

Our feature stories are about how to live better in the new era of longevity, the ancient art of Yang Sheng, and the benefits of castor oil. Wellness friends from around the world have provided tips for ageing well. We look at the impact of emotions on a long, healthy life, what it means to be whole-listic, wellness and ageing with a 'real life Thelma and Louise', energetic acceptance, and pinpoint the location of the elusive fountain of youth.

Our interview features showcase amazing stories from Prema Joy and Laura Gindac, who share insights into their journey to discovering their pathway to becoming wellness advocates. We delve into why self-care is a necessity for healthy ageing and your hormones, and the importance of self-care and establishing boundaries. Reclaiming your life force with Qi Gong, an illuminating journey with long COVID, and why cortisol is a double-edged sword.

We explore five keys to travelling well, resistance training, the Alexander Technique, and the role of gut health. We learn how to successfully embrace pro-ageing by nurturing your skin, and empower our confidence with permanent cosmetics. We also revisit a 30-year-old favourite with our film review, our wellness activity helps you to find ways to incorporate movement in your day, and there's sign-up links to our programs and a link to our free breathe meditation.

Thank you for being here! We love creating this magazine and trust that you will enjoy everything we've included as much as we do.

Stay well.

Natalie Pickett

Entrepreneur, Speaker, Mentor

Join the 'Wellness on Time' community

Visit us online:
www.wellnessontime.com

Follow us on Facebook:
https://www.facebook.com/wellnessontime

Follow us on Instagram:
https://www.instagram.com/wellnessontime

LinkedIn: https://www.linkedin.com/company/wellness-on-time

Wellness on Time Magazine

Issue 6

In this issue ...

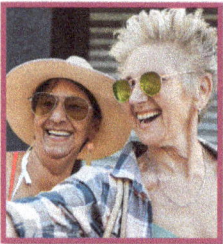
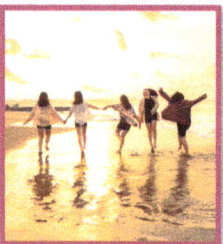

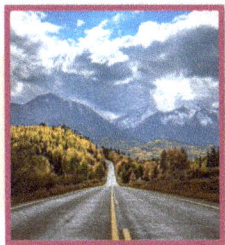

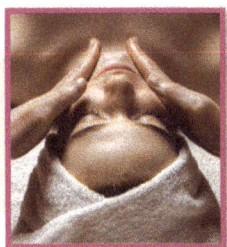

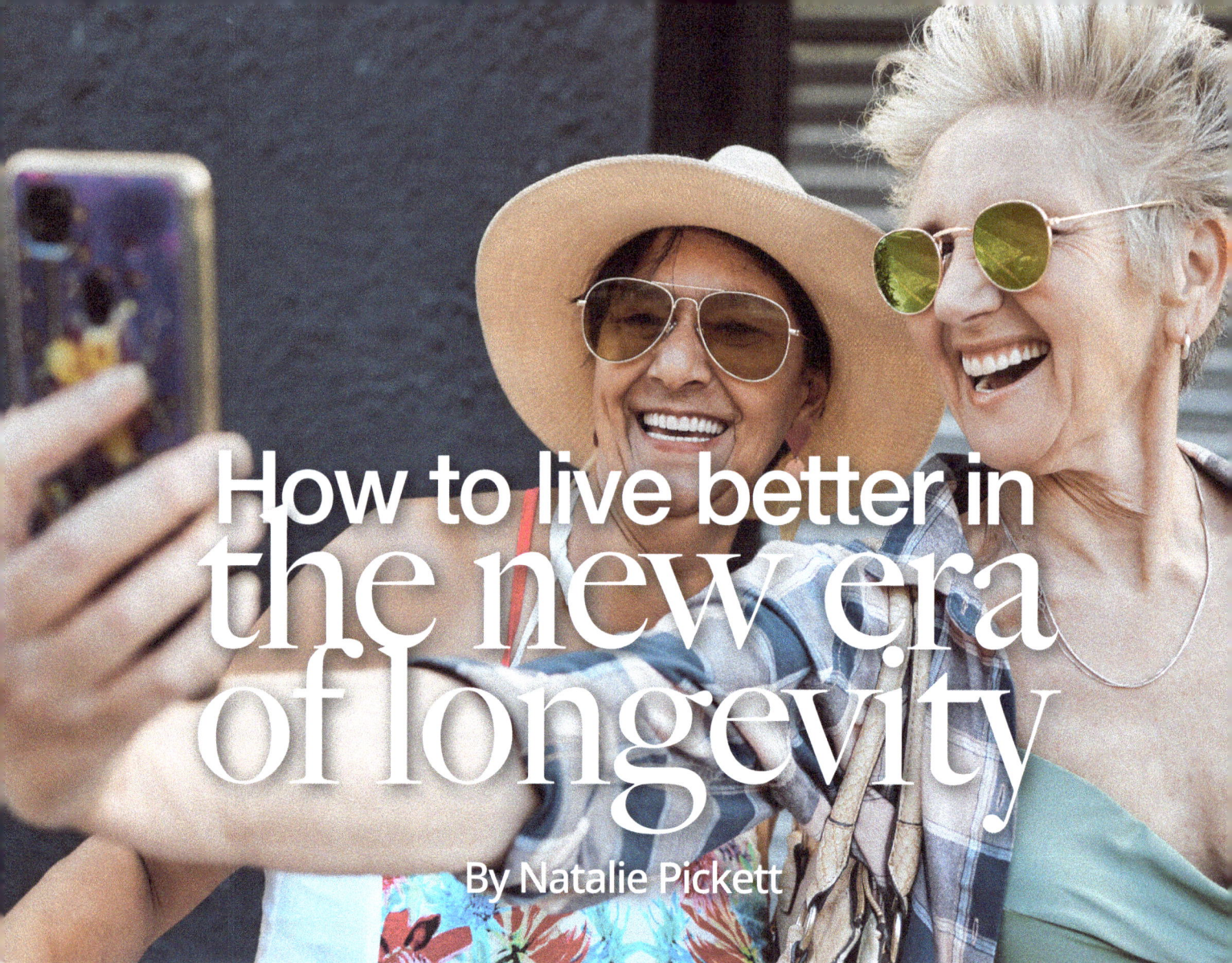

How to live better in the new era of longevity

By Natalie Pickett

As we journey further into the 21st Century, advances in medicine, technology, and choices about how we travel through life are transforming our understanding of ageing. Over the past century, global life expectancy has surged dramatically. In the early 1900s, the average lifespan was just around 47 years. Today, many people in developed countries can expect to live well into their 80s or even beyond. This shift prompts not just a longer life, but a richer, more fulfilling one. The question now is 'How can we optimise our well-being in this new era?'.

It's a funny thing. When we're children, we get excited about getting older and eagerly await each birthday – proudly telling people how old we are as part of our social introduction. At some point, this changes, and age is no longer mentioned; 'Please don't ask my age', or 'Never ask a lady her age'. People say they don't want to get older, but the alternative to not getting older means we are no longer here. We even have terms like 'anti-ageing', which is really more about how to stay young in how we look and feel.

The term 'longevity' refers to a long life, but it's important to differentiate between mere existence and quality of life. Living longer shouldn't mean merely surviving, it should mean thriving. The focus is shifting from how long we live to how well we live, with an emphasis on our health, happiness, and fulfillment.

> The focus is shifting from how long we live to how well we live, with an emphasis on our health, happiness, and fulfillment.

Research in gerontology has unveiled fascinating insights into the ageing process. Factors such as genetics, environment, lifestyle, and social connections play crucial roles in determining not only how long we live, but how well we age.

In their research, Italian demographer Gianni Pes and his colleague Michel Poulain discovered that Sardinia had an unusually high concentration of centenarians. Realising that this was significant, they looked for other areas with similar longevity statistics, marking the locations on a map with blue dots. They coined the term 'Blue Zones' to describe regions where people live notably longer and healthier lives.

Dan Buettner, an explorer, author, and National Geographic Fellow, later expanded this concept, conducting extensive research in these areas. In 2004, he mapped five key Blue Zones – Sardinia (Italy), Okinawa (Japan), Nicoya Peninsula (Costa Rica), Ikaria (Greece), and Loma Linda (California, USA). His work highlights the unique lifestyle characteristics that contribute to the longevity of their inhabitants, emphasising the importance of diet, social engagement, and a sense of purpose, ultimately offering valuable lessons on how to cultivate a healthier, more fulfilling life.

Learning from those who lived well is something I try to embrace. I can remember reading an article some years ago about Jeanne Calment, from France, who lived to be 122. Mme Calment said 'I've never had to face anything that could make me lose my temper. I'm not afraid of anything, even of dying. I'm too old to worry!' ... and this one I've always remembered 'I took pleasure whenever I could!' Emma Morano from Italy, who lived to be 117, was quoted as saying 'I eat what I like, and I don't worry too much. The secret is to be happy and stay true to yourself.' My takeaway from these valuable observations was the importance of doing things that bring joy and savouring life's special moments.

Sometimes life is stressful, but worry is wasteful. Take action to solve the things you need to, but overthinking, and worry helps no one.

Kameo Matsumoto from Okinawa in Japan's Blue Zone lived to be 107 and said, 'Stay active, stay curious, and never lose your sense of wonder about the world.' I love this – maintaining a sense of wonder, stay curious, keep learning, and explore!

In Australia, Irene Eadie, who celebrated her 105th birthday before passing away in 2023, attributed her longevity in part to her love of dancing. She took up dancing in her 70s, which she credited as a significant factor in her longevity and happiness. She emphasised the joy and physical activity that dancing brought to her life. In interviews she said 'I've lived long because I've always enjoyed the simple things – gardening, a good book, and my family around me. But dancing has been a big part of my life too; it keeps you young at heart!'. Her late start in dancing showcases the idea that it's never too late to adopt new activities that promote health and well-being.

I used to prioritise everything else but my joy, putting off fun activities until the 'work' was done. Changing my focus to 'follow my joy' created a big shift. I now encourage others to do the same in my writing, speaking and mentoring businesses. Life should be fun, and our work and business should be too!

Anita Moorjani, who was diagnosed with lymphoma that sent her health into a critical state, experienced a profound near-death experience while in a coma. She reported feeling an overwhelming sense of peace and love, gaining insight into her life and the nature of existence. After making a miraculous recovery, she dedicated her life to sharing her story. Her book, *Dying to Be Me*, emphasises that embracing who we truly are and loving ourselves is crucial for healing and fulfillment. Realising that she had spent most of her life focusing on fear and expectations of others, one of her key insights is encapsulated in her quote 'To love yourself is to recognise that you are not only worthy of love but also capable of it'. This reflects her understanding of self-love and acceptance that emerged from her transformative experience.

Understand your core values and what is important to you. Create a focus of what you want and don't be concerned about what others think.

> Understand your core values and what is important to you. Create a focus of what you want and don't be concerned about what others think.

Genetics does come into play, but that doesn't necessarily lock us into certain health outcomes as we age. In his book *Meta Human*, Deepak Chopra asserts 'You are not just a physical body. You are not just a mind. You are not just a collection of habits. You are a possibility.' He emphasises that while our genes and DNA play a role in our health, they account for only about 5% of our overall well-being. This highlights the transformative power of lifestyle choices and environmental factors, which can influence the remaining 95%. Chopra advocates for a holistic approach that transcends genetic determinism, empowering individuals to shape their health through conscious choices, mindfulness, and self-awareness. This perspective invites us to see ageing not merely as a biological process, but as an opportunity for transformation and growth. By embracing the potential within us, we can redefine our lives.

Lessons in longevity from the Blue Zones

Nearly everything we see related to our health emphasises diet, and yes, the food we eat is important. One consistent feature of the Blue Zones is not just what people eat – nutrient-dense whole foods, and home-cooked meals – but also the sense of connection and community surrounding food. People cook together, eat together, and celebrate together.

On the island of Ikaria, beverages play a significant role, particularly herbal teas made from sage and rosemary. As the birthplace of Dionysus, the Greek god of wine, there is a long history of winemaking here, and I was delighted to discover that the inhabitants credited wine as a key factor in their longevity! Once again, this was a savoured experience enjoyed with friends.

Regular physical activity was a hallmark across all Blue Zones, with people moving naturally throughout their day. For some, this involved their work; for others, it was the challenge of navigating steep village streets. Community involvement through dance and sports – like the current craze of pickleball – also encouraged physical activity.

Rest is another important strategy, highlighted by the practice of afternoon naps, which help reduce stress and improve overall health.

Okinawa boasts the world's highest concentration of female centenarians. A strong sense of purpose, often referred to as "ikigai," is a key element of their longevity. Additionally, sitting on the floor rather than chairs and frequently getting up and down fosters movement and improves balance. These women emphasise the importance of having fun, asserting that laughter brings longevity! Loneliness can also be an issue for older individuals, but this is addressed through strong family and community ties. There is a sincere focus on looking out for one another, which is considered a core value. It's clear that keeping minds engaged is essential, with the community honouring and revering the wisdom and values of their elders.

Stress less – worry does nothing for you. Ageing is not something to hide or ignore; longevity is not a chore, it's a joyful journey.

> Stress less – worry does nothing for you. Ageing is not something to hide or ignore; longevity is not a chore, it's a joyful journey.

Creating a longevity mindset

Embracing the age of longevity requires a shift in mindset. Here are my key strategies to foster a longevity-oriented lifestyle:

1. **Cultivate relationships** Strong social connections are one of the most significant predictors of longevity. Building and maintaining relationships can enhance emotional support, reduce stress, and foster a sense of belonging. Whether through family, friends, or community groups, prioritising these connections is essential.

2. **Stay active and engaged** Physical and mental activities are vital for maintaining health and cognitive function. Engaging in hobbies, volunteering, or joining clubs not only keeps you active, but also provides opportunities for social interaction.

3. **Prioritise sleep** Quality sleep is crucial for overall health, because it is widely acknowledged for enhancing cognitive function, emotional regulation, and physical health. Developing a consistent sleep schedule and creating a restful environment can improve sleep quality.

4. **Embrace lifelong learning** Curiosity and the pursuit of knowledge can keep the mind sharp. Whether through formal education, reading, or exploring new skills, lifelong learning stimulates cognitive function and can provide a sense of purpose.

5. **Practice mindfulness** Incorporating mindfulness practices such as meditation and deep-breathing exercises can help reduce stress and promote mental well-being. Mindfulness encourages a positive outlook on life and enhances emotional resilience.

6. **Harnessing technology for health** Technology plays an integral role in enhancing our lives in the age of longevity. Wearable devices, telemedicine, and health apps allow us to monitor our health, track our fitness goals, and stay connected with healthcare providers. Innovations in biotechnology are also paving the way for personalised medicine, targeting individual needs, and optimising our health outcomes.

7. **The role of preventive care** In the longevity equation, preventive healthcare is crucial. Regular check-ups, and screenings can help catch potential health issues early, allowing for timely intervention. Health education and awareness can empower individuals to take charge of their health proactively.

As part of having a good life, the idea of an equally good death encompasses the notion of passing away with dignity, comfort, and a sense of closure. Engaging in open conversations with loved ones about end-of-life wishes is essential, as it ensures that your desires regarding care, comfort, and even final arrangements are acknowledged and respected. These discussions can alleviate the burden on family members during a difficult time, allowing them to honour your preferences. Additionally, having your financial affairs in order, such as Wills, insurance policies, and any other necessary legal documents, provides peace-of-mind for you and your loved ones. By proactively addressing these aspects, you create an environment where you can pass away peacefully, knowing that your wishes are clear, and your family is supported.

The age of longevity presents unprecedented opportunities to redefine what it means to age. By adopting a holistic approach to health through focusing on physical, mental, and social well-being, we can not only extend our years, but also enrich the quality of our lives.

> By adopting a holistic approach to health through focusing on physical, mental, and social well-being, we can not only extend our years, but also enrich the quality of our lives.

Embracing this new paradigm means understanding that ageing is not a decline, but each stage a phase of life filled with potential. As we navigate this journey, let us commit to living better, cultivating joy, and fostering connections that enhance our experience in this exciting new age.

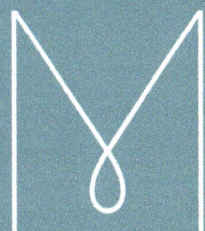
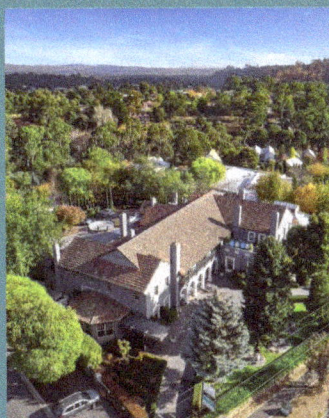 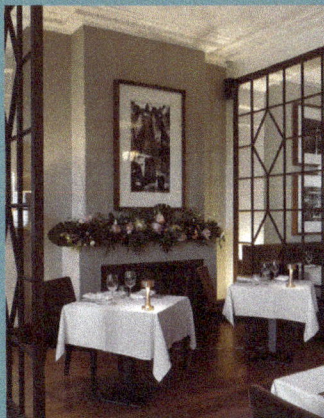 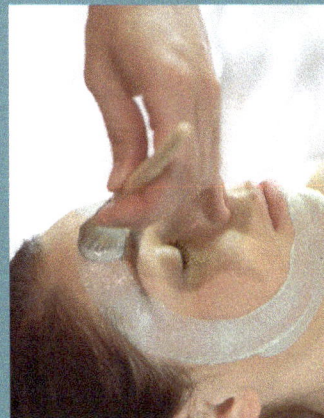

Tips for ageing well

We asked some of our wellness friends from around the world to share their top tips on ageing well.

Wellness on Time Founder, Natalie Pickett, says 'The older I get, the more convinced I am that ageing well is more about how we feel rather than how we look. Having experienced chronic pain more than once in my life, I know that when we don't feel well in our body, we feel older than we are. If our energy is depleted, nurturing ourselves and taking time to restore our energy and getting our being in balance is vital. A being in harmony is connected through mind, body, soul, heart, and spirit. We spend our lives with a focus on 'doing' rather than 'being', and there can be feelings of guilt when we are doing nothing – yet in the 'nothing' is the key to restoring our energy. This can be as simple as a sitting quietly with a cup of tea, a daily nap or meditation, massage, spa treatments and acupuncture. Spending time re-connecting with nature and engaging all of the senses is a 'go to' for me. Once restored, I can make time for play and do things that bring me joy, which includes precious time with friends, social activities, dance, sports, or my favourite wellness modalities such as Feldenkrais, yoga, or pilates.'

Chantel Ryan, The Minimalist Naturopath says 'Ageing well isn't about doing more, it's about doing less, but with intention. Focus on simplifying your environment, routines, and even your thoughts. Decluttering your living space can reduce stress and create a calming atmosphere. Paring down your daily habits to just what nourishes you – physically, emotionally, and mentally – frees up energy for what truly matters. Minimalism isn't just a lifestyle, it's a pathway to graceful ageing by keeping only what sustains your vitality.'

> Paring down your daily habits to just what nourishes you – physically, emotionally, and mentally – frees up energy for what truly matters.

Editor-in-chief of *Yorkshire Women's Life* (UK), and Mental Health Campaigner Dawn-Maria France stressed 'The importance of taking care of your body with a healthy diet along with regular check-ups with your doctor for early issue detection. Equally crucial is staying active and maintaining social connections for mental well-being. Nurture strong relationships and engage in social activities to stay active and vibrant!'

Chloe Jane, Cosmetic Registered Nurse from By Golden says 'Embracing your natural beauty and feeling confident within your skin is the first step. Healthy skin is the new in; it's the biggest organ in your body and it's the first thing people see when they look at you. Your skin tells the story of your life – it shows your repeated emotions (in fine lines and wrinkles, smile and frown lines). It shows years spent in the sun at the beach, and it shows your trauma in your scars. Ageing gracefully is allowing the world to see the beautiful life you lived through your skin, whilst keeping it healthy, hydrated and volumised. Allow your skin to be the example of how you love and care for yourself. Minimising years of sun damage and pigmentation through Sun Protection Factor (SPF) and laser therapies, as well as replacing volume loss, can show the love and care you gave yourself in the younger years.'

Cleveland OH, Facial Plastic Surgeon Dr Diana Ponsky suggested that 'Ageing is inevitable and universal. Although genetics definitely plays a role, ageing well is about embracing and anticipating the natural changes that come with time. We are living longer, thanks to improvements in health awareness. Consistent skincare, including daily use of sunscreen and moisturisers, is essential to protect and nourish the skin. Regular exercise, a balanced diet, and staying hydrated play crucial roles in maintaining a youthful appearance. Additionally, there are non-invasive treatments that can enhance natural beauty, such as dermal fillers or laser therapies, to refresh and rejuvenate. Sometimes, a little 'nip and tuck' can help bridge the gap that exercise alone and/or genetics cannot achieve. Ultimately, ageing well is about feeling good in your own skin and enjoying each stage of life with grace and positivity.'

Jess Patra, Spiritual Mentor and Breathwork practitioner and Founder of Putu Jess Patra tells us that the secret recipe to ageing well is 'A daily practice of conscious connected breathwork and meditation. Activities like breathwork and meditation regulate your nervous system, reduce stress and calm the mind.'

Daisy Cabral, CEO of Bella All Natural says 'Ageing well isn't about looking like a million bucks – it's about feeling great from the inside out. Sure, exercise, good food, and sleep are your basic building blocks, but don't forget about having fun and staying connected. Keep your brain active, make time for friends, and find something that gets you excited. And hey, it's never too late to start! Small steps make a big difference. Listen to your body, take care of yourself, and enjoy the ride. Ageing is a natural part of life, so let's make it a good one!'

Cristina Dovan, Writer, and Life Mindset Transformation Coach, based in the UK told us 'Everyone talks about ageing, but most of them focus on aesthetics. For me, wellness is about having a holistic approach to mind, body, and spirit. We also need to take care of our mind – what we let in and what we consume. If we consume toxic information, our life will reflect that, and we will find ourselves involved in toxic situations more easily. Changing our 'fixed' mindset to a 'growth' mindset by expanding our minds and constantly learning is key. Many people think "I'm getting old so it's natural that my health declines". You are harming yourself by influencing your brain in a negative way without even knowing it. Our brain doesn't register the difference between what is real and what is not, so feed it positive information! Tell yourself you feel young and live a life that keeps you young at heart and mind.'

> Our brain doesn't register the difference between what is real and what is not, so feed it positive information! Tell yourself you feel young and live a life that keeps you young at heart and mind.

Megan Hayward, Founder of Mimi Moon Meno, shared that 'In Australia, there are around 80,000 women per year entering their menopause journey, and that women continue to be over-represented in several major health concerns. The best way women can prepare for perimenopause, mid-life and beyond is to adopt my 'Movement, Mindset, Modify' mantra. Modify for the hormonal fluctuations of perimenopause and accept the things you are not in control of – let them go. Have the courage to take control of what you can. I suggest reviewing what is no longer serving you positively and make a change.'

Eugenie Pepper, Psychotherapist, Clinical Hypnotherapist and Counseller suggests 'Meditation, hypnosis, and mindfulness can help you age well by reducing stress, improving focus, promoting relaxation, enhancing emotional well-being, and fostering positive behaviour change. To incorporate these techniques into your routine, start with short sessions and gradually increase the duration. Try to find a quiet space free from distractions, and focus on your breath during meditation. Consider working with a certified hypnotherapist. Practice mindfulness throughout the day by staying present. Engage in mindful breathing and gratitude exercises. Attend classes or workshops to deepen your practice and connect with others. Consistent practice and a positive attitude can help support a healthy body and mind as you age.'

Jane Langof, Feng Shui Master and Author of *Feng Shui, A Homeowner's Guide to Abundance*, suggested that 'Ageing well is about creating harmony within and around you, and this starts with the spaces you inhabit. By designing your home to support your health and vitality, you can naturally promote better sleep, reduce stress, and foster a sense of well-being. Feng Shui principles can help balance the energy in your home with elements like soft lighting, serene colours, and clutter-free environments enhancing calm and reducing stress, which are important for ageing well. A well-organised space for easy movement and social interaction encourages an active lifestyle, which is essential for maintaining physical and mental health. Your surroundings are an extension of yourself, and by creating positive energy in your space you can support a happier, healthier life that keeps you feeling more vibrant and youthful.'

Fiona Maria, Singing Facilitator and Founder of Sing High Sing Low tells us that 'Singing is a wonderful tool for staying healthy as we age, because it brings physical and mental health benefits. Singing improves lung capacity, boosts cardiovascular health, and strengthens our core muscles. Importantly, it's a 'whole brain' activity, a great cognitive workout (activating 10 areas across our brain) and helping to keep our brain sharp. When we sing, all the 'feel good' hormones – oxytocin, serotonin, dopamine – are released and cortisol levels drop. Singing simultaneously reduces stress, soothes anxiety, and enhances our mood. Singing with others is where the real magic happens! It brings a sense of community, and counters loneliness. It is also free and has no side effects! Don't think about perfection or performance, just about joining in. Everyone has a voice and using it in a 'singing kind of a way' is a proven effective step in ageing well.'

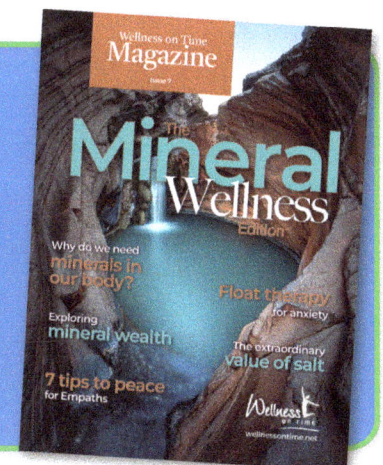

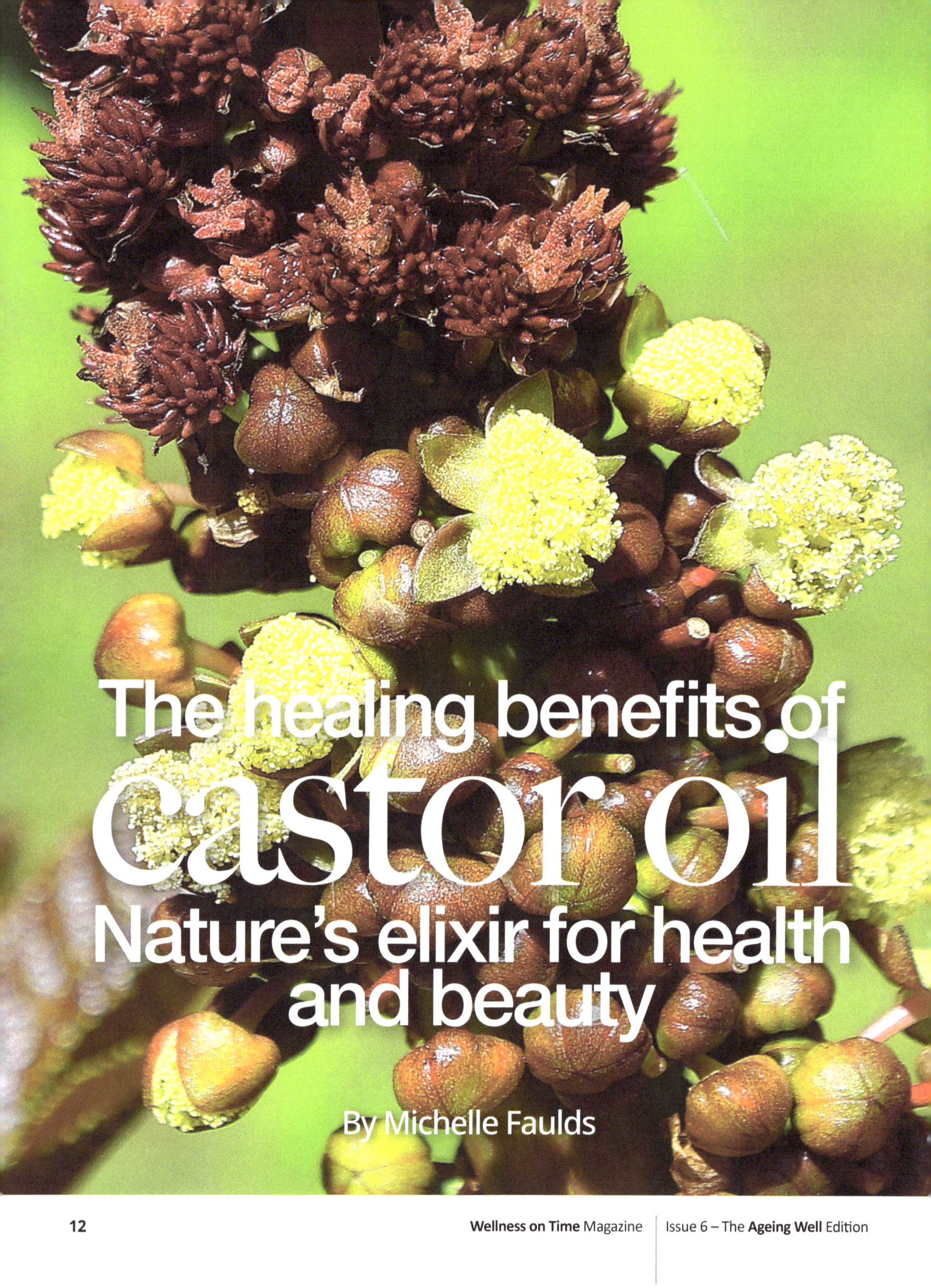

The healing benefits of
castor oil
Nature's elixir for health and beauty

By Michelle Faulds

In an age where wellness and natural health are becoming paramount, more people are turning to ancient remedies to rejuvenate their bodies and skin. Among these time-tested solutions, castor oil stands out as a versatile elixir with a multitude of healing benefits. I have used castor oil in my own healing journey to assist with fertility and inflammation. I was able to conceive in my first IVF round at age 48, and lost a whopping 100 pounds! Let's explore a few reasons why this humble oil should be a staple in your wellness and beauty routine.

Castor oil is derived from the seeds of the *Ricinus communis* plant (pictured). Its use dates to ancient Egypt, where it was revered for its medicinal properties. The therapeutic potential of castor oil lies in its unique composition; it is rich in ricinoleic acid, a fatty acid known for its anti-inflammatory and antimicrobial properties.

It is important to appreciate that not all castor oils are created equal. When selecting castor oil, it's crucial to choose organic and hexane-free varieties. Organic castor oil ensures that the product is free from pesticides and harmful chemicals, which can compromise its purity and efficacy. Hexane, a solvent used in oil extraction, can leave toxic residues if not properly removed. Therefore, opting for hexane-free castor oil guarantees a cleaner, safer product.

The extraction method also significantly impacts the quality of castor oil. Cold-pressed castor oil is made by pressing the seeds without using heat, preserving the oil's natural nutrients and active compounds. In contrast, expeller-pressed oil involves heat during extraction, which can degrade the beneficial properties of the oil. For the highest quality and potency, cold-pressed castor oil is the superior choice.

Health benefits

1. Natural laxative

One of the most well-known uses of castor oil is as a natural laxative. A small dose of this oil can stimulate the bowels and provide relief from constipation. Its effectiveness is backed by science, making it a reliable option for those seeking a natural solution to digestive issues.

2. Anti-inflammatory and pain relief

Castor oil's high ricinoleic acid content gives it powerful anti-inflammatory properties. When applied topically using a castor oil pack, it can reduce inflammation and provide pain relief for sore muscles and joints. This makes it an excellent remedy for conditions like arthritis and muscle aches.

3. Boosts immune function

Castor oil packs applied to the skin are believed to enhance the body's lymphatic system. This system plays a crucial role in detoxification and immune function. By promoting lymphatic drainage, castor oil can help boost your body's natural defence mechanisms.

Beauty benefits

1. Moisturising Castor oil is an excellent moisturiser due to its high fatty acid content, which helps to lock in moisture. It can be particularly beneficial for dry and flaky skin, leaving it soft and hydrated. Simply massage a few drops into your skin to reap its moisturising benefits.

2. Hair growth Castor oil is widely used as a natural remedy for hair growth. Its nourishing properties can strengthen hair follicles and promote thicker, healthier hair. Apply it to your scalp and leave it on overnight for the best results.

3. Treating acne Thanks to its antimicrobial properties, castor oil can help reduce acne and prevent future breakouts. Apply a small amount to the affected area before bed and rinse off in the morning for clearer skin.

4. Strengthening nails If you struggle with brittle nails, castor oil can help. Its hydrating properties can strengthen your nails and prevent them from breaking. Massage a small amount into your nails and cuticles daily for noticeable improvement.

Incorporating organic, hexane-free, cold-pressed castor oil into your wellness and beauty regimen has been known to yield numerous benefits. From promoting digestive health to enhancing your skin and hair, this versatile oil is a natural powerhouse. For those passionate about natural health and beauty, castor oil is a must-have in your arsenal.

> Incorporating organic, hexane-free, cold-pressed castor oil into your wellness and beauty regimen has been known to yield numerous benefits. From promoting digestive health to enhancing your skin and hair, this versatile oil is a natural powerhouse.

Are you ready to experience the healing benefits of castor oil? Make sure you choose the highest quality to ensure optimal results. Transform your health and beauty routine today with castor oil – nature's elixir for health and beauty.

Michelle Faulds is the President of Healing Haven, an online health and wellness store providing natural alternative health products.

Take time to breathe

We took our first breath to enter this world. We can go for days without food and water, but only minutes without breath. Many of us are not breathing properly.

Good breathing helps us to relax, regulates our system, supplies oxygen to our cells and our brain. Many of us shallow breathe when we are stressed, and often by the end of the day many of us are shallow breathing. Take some time to concentrate on your breathing. Gentle slow breaths right down into your belly.

Scan our QR code to access our free 'Wellness on Time' belly breathing meditation

Save 15% with coupon code CASTOR15

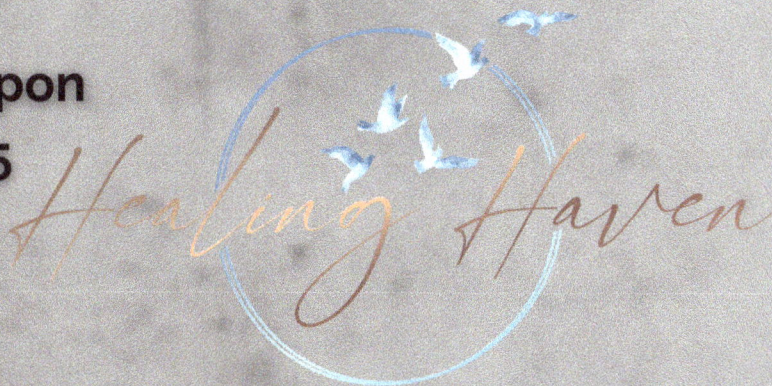

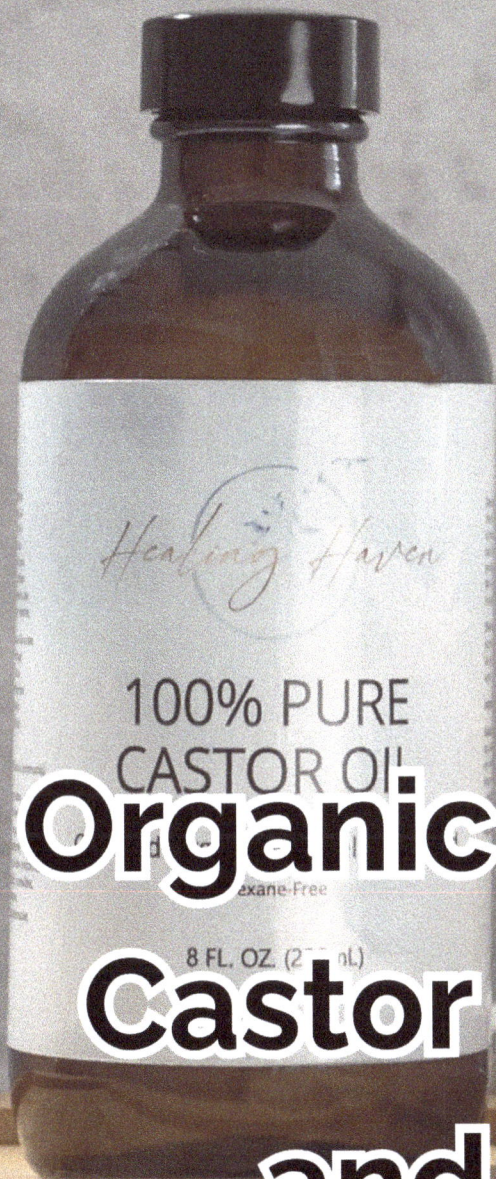

Healing Haven

100% PURE CASTOR OIL

8 FL. OZ. (250 mL)

Organic Castor Oil Castor Oil Packs and more!

www.healinghavenshop.com

Yang Sheng
The ancient art of nourishing life

By Dr Nicola Macdonald

'Yang Sheng' – an ancient Chinese philosophy – centres on the idea of 'nourishment of life'. This holistic approach to health and well-being emphasises the importance of maintaining balance within the body, mind, and spirit to achieve longevity, prevent illness, and enhance the quality of life. Rooted in Traditional Chinese Medicine (TCM), Taoism, and Confucianism, Yang Sheng has evolved over centuries into a comprehensive system of self-care practices that promote overall health.

Historical background

Yang Sheng's origins can be traced back to ancient Chinese texts, most notably the 'Huangdi Neijing' (The Yellow Emperor's Inner Canon), a foundational work of TCM from the 3rd Century BCE. These early writings emphasise living in harmony with nature and understanding the body's rhythms as key to maintaining health. Central to Yang Sheng is the concept of 'Qi' (气), the vital life force that flows through all living beings. In TCM, the harmonious flow of Qi is essential for good health, while its blockage or imbalance can lead to illness. Yang Sheng practices are designed to ensure the smooth flow of Qi, thereby preventing disease and promoting vitality.

Core principles of Yang Sheng

1. Balance and harmony A fundamental principle of Yang Sheng is achieving balance and harmony within the body and with the external environment. This balance is often discussed in terms of Yin and Yang, the opposing but complementary forces that exist in all things. Yin represents qualities such as cold, passivity, and darkness, while Yang embodies heat, activity, and light. Health is believed to result from a harmonious balance between Yin and Yang.

2. Prevention over cure Yang Sheng places a strong emphasis on preventing illness rather than treating it after the fact. This proactive approach involves regular self-care practices that strengthen the body's natural defences, making it more resilient to disease. This philosophy aligns with the TCM adage, '... treating the root, not just the symptoms', which encourages addressing the underlying causes of health issues before they manifest.

3. Adaptation to nature Living in harmony with nature is a cornerstone of Yang Sheng. This principle involves adapting one's lifestyle to the changing seasons, climate, and environmental conditions. For instance, eating seasonal foods, choosing clothing to suit the weather, and modifying daily routines to align with natural rhythms are all practices that support health and well-being.

4. Moderation Moderation in all aspects of life is crucial in Yang Sheng. Whether it's diet, exercise, work, or even emotions, over-indulgence or deficiency can disrupt the body's balance, leading to health problems. Yang Sheng advocates for a balanced approach, where moderation ensures that all aspects of life are in harmony.

5. Cultivation of the mind and spirit Mental and spiritual health are considered just as important as physical health in Yang Sheng. Practices such as meditation, mindfulness, and breathing exercises (like Qigong and Tai Chi) are used to calm the mind, reduce stress, and cultivate inner peace. A tranquil mind is believed to foster a healthy body, as emotional imbalances can disrupt the flow of Qi and lead to physical ailments.

Practices of Yang Sheng

1. Diet A balanced diet of natural, whole foods is a cornerstone of Yang Sheng. Emphasis is placed on the consumption of fresh vegetables, fruits, whole grains, and lean proteins. The diet should be adjusted according to the seasons, with warming foods in winter and cooling foods in summer. Mindful eating practices, such as eating slowly and in a relaxed environment, are also encouraged as they contribute to better digestion and overall health.

2. Exercise Regular physical activity is essential, but it is important that exercise is done in moderation and in harmony with one's individual constitution and environment. Traditional Chinese exercises like Tai Chi and Qigong are highly recommended because they combine physical movement with breath control and mental focus, promoting the smooth flow of Qi throughout the body.

3. Breathing techniques Proper breathing is believed to directly influence the flow of Qi. Techniques such as deep abdominal breathing and controlled breath exercises are used to enhance lung capacity and reduce stress. These practices are often integrated into physical exercises like Qigong and Tai Chi, further enhancing their benefits.

4. Sleep and rest Adequate rest and quality sleep are vital components of Yang Sheng. The body's Qi is replenished during sleep, making it a critical period for healing and rejuvenation. Yang Sheng advises against overstimulation before bedtime, advocates for a regular sleep schedule, and emphasises the importance of creating a restful environment to ensure deep, restorative sleep.

5. Emotional regulation Yang Sheng encourages the regulation of emotions through practices such as mindfulness, meditation, and maintaining a positive outlook on life. Emotional imbalances, such as excessive anger, sadness, or anxiety, can disrupt the flow of Qi and lead to health problems. By cultivating emotional resilience, we can maintain our mental and physical health.

6. Environmental harmony Clean air, a peaceful living space, and connection with nature are considered essential for maintaining health. Feng Shui, the practice of arranging living spaces to promote harmony and positive energy flow, is often incorporated into Yang Sheng practices.

Modern applications of Yang Sheng

In the modern world, Yang Sheng has gained popularity as a holistic approach to health and well-being. People are turning to these ancient practices as a way to manage stress, improve mental clarity, and maintain physical health in a fast-paced society. Many contemporary wellness practices, such as mindfulness, yoga, and clean eating, share similarities with Yang Sheng principles. By integrating these practices into daily life, individuals can achieve a balanced and harmonious balance state, leading to improved health and longevity.

Dr Nicola Macdonald is a Chinese Medicine Practitioner, Hatha Yoga Teacher, Retreat Host, Creator of the AcuHarmonics system and Founder of Health Connect Shen.

How your emotions have an impact on living a long and healthy life

By Prema Joy

When you make your new year's resolutions around health, what are the things you decide? 'I'll join a gym ... lose 10lbs ... eat healthier ... walk, exercise more ... take up mindfulness and meditation'? It's unusual for us to say, 'I'm going to work on my emotional health', right?

And yet, extensive research by the Centers for Disease Control and Prevention (CDC) reveals that over 85% of illnesses are emotionally based, influenced by suppressing or avoiding our instinctive emotional response to life's challenges.

We have been conditioned to believe that being healthy is about fitness, energy, and mindfulness. Whilst focusing on one or all of these things is beneficial, we do not often give any credit to our emotions for a long and healthy life.

Many people are not aware of how to safely feel an emotion in their body. Depending on our culture, family life and beliefs, we think some emotions are good and ok, and some are bad and not ok to feel. Because of this, many people are 'numbed out', addicted to substances, workaholics, abusive, depressed, and on medication to make them feel better.

We all have a thing called a 'biological imperative' – a drive to survive, grow, maintain – and without it, we wouldn't be here as individuals or a species. For that to happen, we also have an awareness within our environment, body, and self, if we are under threat.

Research by the celebrated American neuroscientist Candace Pert, identified that when our emotions are expressed and flow freely, they last for approximately 30–60 seconds, and '... all systems are united and made whole'.[1]

When we are in harmony, our biological imperative moves to grow, sustain and maintain. We feel in love with life, we connect with others, our immune system is working, and we relax on the inside.

When they are repressed, denied, or not allowed for whatever reason, they become blocked, the cell receptors shut down and are susceptible to disease. We disconnect and focus on the threats in life.

Many people have suffered some form of emotional shut down in childhood – being humiliated, bullied, left out, victimised – and some even traumatised by divorce, abuse, war, or a parent dying.

We learned to deal with our emotions by either shutting them down, being distracted, (food, games, drugs, alcohol), projecting and blaming others (violent outbursts), analysing them (anxiousness), or wallowing in them (telling a story and reliving it). We learned from our parents and their behavioural model.

My mum's approach to comforting me involved offering food to soothe my emotions. When I had a bad day at school, rather than allowing me to feel sad, she would encourage me to have a treat like a biscuit or cake to feel better. This stemmed from her own experiences during the war when she was 7, where she found comfort in a small square of chocolate given to her nightly in an air raid shelter. This upbringing taught me to suppress my feelings and emotionally eat, resulting in struggles with my weight for most of my life.

Emotions are a natural healthy automatic release in the body. When we shut them down, repress, analyse, project, wallow, or distract ourselves from them, we are not feeling them.

Feeling our feelings is easy. It can be uncomfortable, because of our conditioning and resistance, but when we do open into a feeling and release it naturally, there is often another feeling underneath. When we can release them all and we are 'empty', there is peace, space, an expansiveness, and when we surrender, our emotions become the gateway to our source.

> When we can release them all and we are 'empty', there is peace, space, an expansiveness, and when we surrender, our emotions become the gateway to our source.

Society's norms dictate which emotions are acceptable, leading many of us to live behind a wall of protection – a mask of 'I'm fine!', which we present to the world to avoid judgement.

We perceive that if we do let go and feel something unwanted – like devastation, rage, or self-hatred – that it will harm us or someone else, or that we may not be able to stop it, and that it confirms us as a bad person. The truth is, if we open and allow a feeling to move through our body naturally, it will diffuse itself, hurting no-one, and because we release it, it doesn't get stored or stuck, and our cell receptors remain open.

Throughout my decades of working with clients, I have helped thousands of people transform their health and lives by allowing their emotions. As for myself, at age 62, having overcome alcoholism, addictions and domestic violence, I am the epitome of a vibrant healthy older woman.

Emotional health is not a luxury – it's a necessity for living a long, healthy life. By prioritising our emotional well-being, we unlock our true potential, our biological imperative stays in 'grow and maintain' and has a positive effect on ourselves and our environment.

Reference

1. Pert, C. (1999). *Molecules of Emotion. The Science Behind Mind Body Medicine: Why You Feel the Way You Feel*. Simon and Schuster, New York.

Prema Joy is an Emotional Healing Expert, Coach and Mentor.

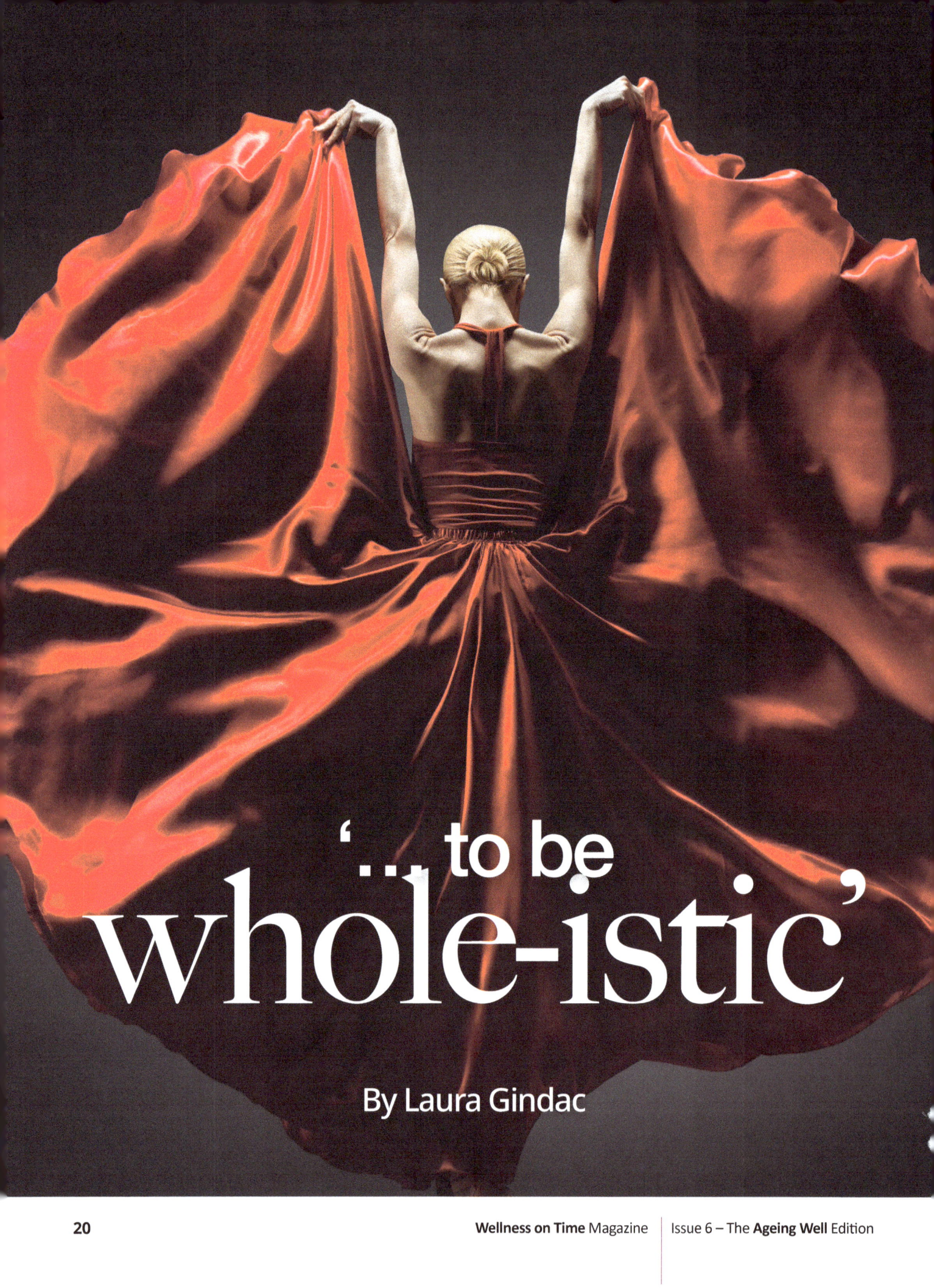

'... to be whole-istic'

By Laura Gindac

Holistic living is often understood as the practice of integrating the physical, emotional, mental, and spiritual aspects of oneself into a harmonious whole. However, the depth of holistic living extends far beyond mere personal well-being – it encompasses how one interacts with and influences the world around them.

At its core, personal holistic practice involves nurturing every facet of your being. This means attending to your physical health through balanced nutrition and exercise, cultivating emotional resilience and mental clarity, and engaging in spiritual practices that align with your values. When you live holistically on an individual level, you seek equilibrium and fulfillment within yourself, striving to be whole and well-rounded.

Teaching holistic living involves sharing these principles with others, often through guidance, counselling, or educational frameworks. This approach emphasises the benefits of holistic practices and aims to inspire others to adopt similar habits and mindsets. The role of a teacher is to illuminate the path and provide tools and wisdom for others to incorporate holistic practices into their lives. While teaching is vital for spreading awareness and understanding, it is inherently a form of external influence.

Being holistic, on the other hand, transcends the act of teaching. It embodies a way of being that permeates every interaction and relationship. When you truly live holistically, you don't merely instruct others on how to achieve balance, you live in such a way that your presence and actions inherently promote harmony and well-being. Your relationships become a reflection of your holistic values, and your interactions are imbued with empathy, respect, and understanding.

The profound difference lies in the essence of embodiment versus dissemination. Teaching holistic principles can influence change, but being holistic means that your life itself becomes a living example of those principles. It's about integrating holistic values into the very fabric of your existence so that every interaction, from the most intimate to the most casual, is a testament to the balance and interconnectedness you strive to cultivate.

In essence, the journey from teaching holistic living to truly being holistic represents a profound evolution. It involves moving from sharing knowledge to embodying and living out the principles in every aspect of life. When one achieves this, their presence and actions can inspire and elevate others, creating a ripple effect that fosters a more harmonious and interconnected world.

Holistic living is like a dance with the Universe, where every step is an exploration of balance and harmony. It's not about achieving a perfect, unblemished existence, but about the gentle art of weaving together your inner and outer worlds. Picture it as a journey along a winding path, where each twist and turn invites you to discover and nurture the many facets of your being.

> Holistic living is like a dance with the Universe, where every step is an exploration of balance and harmony. It's not about achieving a perfect, unblemished existence, but about the gentle art of weaving together your inner and outer worlds.

In this dance, perfection is an elusive star in the night sky. The true beauty lies in our graceful attempts to reach for it, in the continuous practice of aligning your life with your deepest values. Imagine each day as a new canvas, where you paint with the colours of your efforts – sometimes bold, sometimes soft, but always evolving. The strokes may not always be flawless, but they create a rich tapestry of experience and growth.

To live holistically is to embrace this journey with all its imperfections. It's about savouring the process and understanding that the rhythm of life is as much about the pauses and missteps as it is about the harmonious flow. Each moment of striving, each effort to bring balance, is a note in the symphony of your life.

Even when the melody falters or the steps feel uncertain, the practice itself is a testament to your dedication. It's in the ongoing attempt to harmonise your actions with your values that the magic unfolds. The effort, though imperfect, creates a ripple of transformation – not just within yourself but in the world around you. And in this ever-evolving dance, the pursuit of holistic living becomes a beautiful, ongoing celebration of life's intricate and radiant journey.

Laura Gindac is the Founder and Owner of XQ-SLESS, a holistic online wellness support tribe.

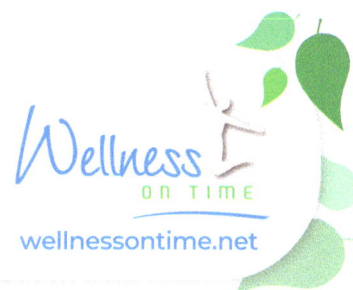

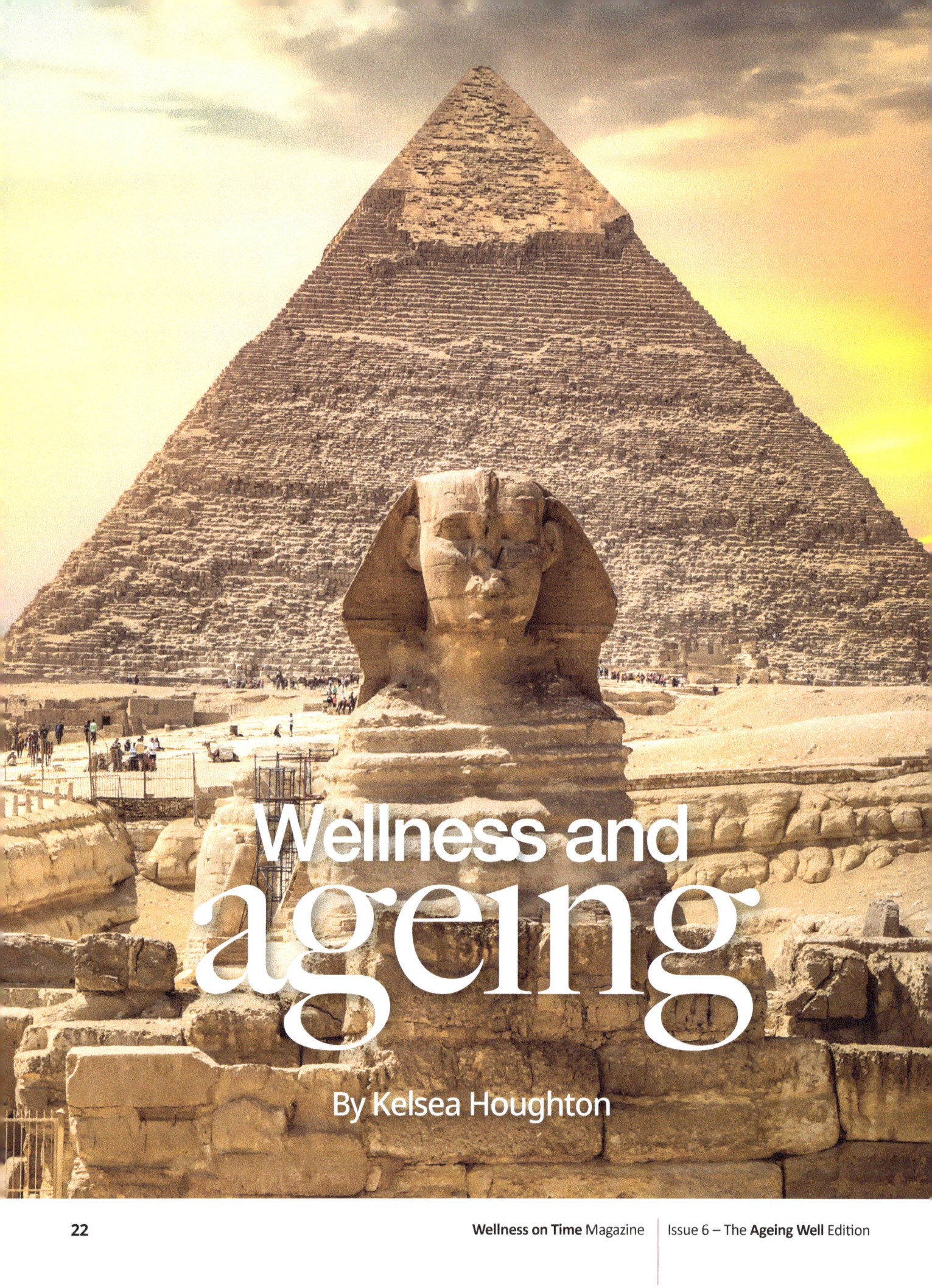

Wellness and ageing

By Kelsea Houghton

Issac Newton might have said it best when he stated, 'A body in motion stays in motion.' Albert Einstein also shared a similar viewpoint in his theory of relativity, identifying that the faster you move in space, the slower you move in time. This theory is so powerful that I have the equation tattooed on the back of my right calf. I've always used it as inspiration towards ageing – a gentle reminder to keep moving and stay young forever. As a lifelong runner and science/math lover, this equation has always had a special place in my heart.

I'll never forget the excitement I would have every morning as a child whenever we stayed with my grandmother or hosted her at our home. Not because she was ready to snuggle and knit all day long like an old woman might've back then, but because she had an amazing morning workout routine, and my brother and I were always eager to be a part of it.

She would stay up late, typically turning in between 11pm and 2am, and sleeping until 9am or so. I'd be sitting in the living room for over an hour anticipating her stirring and coming out of her bedroom dressed in her cotton shorts and tank top, with her small white timer in hand. She'd smile at me and say, 'Are you ready?' – and we would begin. She had a series of exercises – toe touches, wide leg stretches, sit-ups, push-ups, and other types of arms, legs, and ab exercises. She'd set her timer for a minute, and we'd do multiple sets of each in a circuit. This woman basically created high intensity interval training (HIIT)! The only people who were doing HIIT in the 90s were Olympians, and it was far from mainstream exercise. How she got tuned into it, I'll never know.

One Summer, I remember doing leg lifts on the floor with her and my brother, who was having a hard time finishing out the minute. He exasperatedly spurted out, 'Are we done yet?!' … begging for the timer to chime! As soon as he asked, the television advertisement loudly answered, 'You'll **never** be done!' We all burst into laughter as our abs burned, and we finished the remaining seconds before finally being able to rest.

She always inspired me to keep moving, to be active, and to live life with love instead of fear. She loved to sing, give back to her community, travel, and was always in motion. I remember unboxing a package from her, directly from Spain, where inside I found a small black furred bull with a red ribbon around his neck. I was in awe that she had gone so far to see something so ancient and rich. In the Summer of 1963, she had also travelled to Israel to see the Holy Lands, and Egypt to visit the Great Pyramids with her best friend, Thelma. Coincidentally, my grandmother's name was Louise (if you're familiar with the 1991 film, Thelma and Louise, about two best friends). Her actions gave me

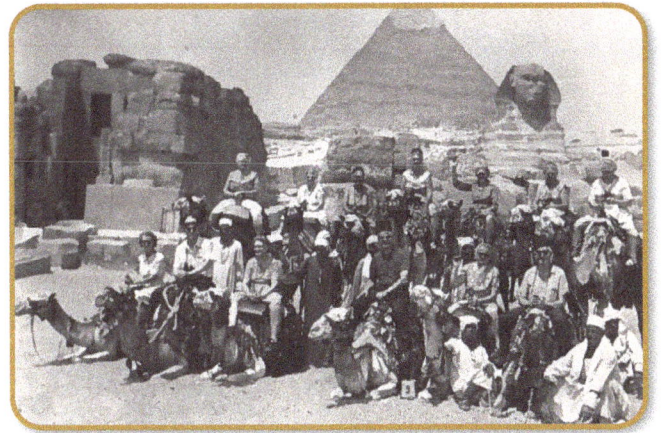

The author's grandmother, Louise (top row, far left), visiting the Great Pyramid in Egypt in the Summer of 1963. Thelma is in the front row, first on the left on a camel.

the courage to travel solo to India for three months when I was 20 years old, and I owe a large part of my adventurous spirit to her.

Fast forward to today, where I am in my thirties, a yoga teacher with extensive training, a great love for travel, and still enjoying a good HIIT session. I live in an area with a large retirement community, and I am easily 25 years younger than anyone else in my local gym classes. I am always humbled as I come out of my 50-minute class, where I huffed and puffed my way through as the 60–85-year-olds complete their sets with steady strength and perseverance. I love this group because it's inspiring and familiar for me, and always reminds me of my own grandmother, who would be kicking my butt right next to me if she were here today.

> I love this group because it's inspiring and familiar for me, and always reminds me of my own grandmother, who would be kicking my butt right next to me if she were here today.

What I can say for sure about our lives, health, and ageing, is that movement of any kind is always positive, and will always benefit us in meeting our longevity with ease, grace, and strength. Not only that, but the way in which we lead our lives goes far beyond our own lifetime, and is naturally instilled in those around us, our children, and grandchildren. I would not have the life I have lived today if not for the strong, loving, and adventurous grandmother I had the honour of knowing and learning from – and those types of long-lasting effects cannot be bought, consumed, or given, **only lived**.

A deep bow to you, my friend. Namaste.

Kelsea Houghton is the Founder of Holistic Hatha Yoga and Creator of Embark on Meditation, Natural Birthing the Yogic Way, and The Path to Inner Peace courses.

Ageing well through *energetic acceptance*

By Casey Castro

Growing older is a journey that we all embark on as we progress through life's stages. But what if we perceived the act of ageing as more than just a slow passage of time? In the esoteric tradition, ageing is viewed as a holy dance with the Universe, providing an opportunity to expand our understanding of ourselves and our connection to the cosmic forces that influence everything. We age gracefully and wisely by practicing energetic acceptance – the ability to embrace internal shifts.

As we age, one of the most difficult problems we face is dealing with the consequences of our decisions. Society teaches us to label these decisions as 'right' or 'wrong', yet this dualistic thinking frequently locks us in a cycle of self-judgement, regret, and resistance. There is no bad or good – there simply just 'is'. Only the route you have chosen exists.

Every decision you've taken has been part of your unique unfolding, bringing you to the lessons and experiences your soul required in this lifetime. The concept of regretting a decision suggests that there is an alternative reality in which a 'better' life exists. However, as we zoom out to examine our lives from a greater perspective, we realise that each twist and turn has been divinely led. We are precisely where we are supposed to be, and every decision we made was the appropriate one for that time.

> Every decision you've taken has been part of your unique unfolding, bringing you to the lessons and experiences your soul required in this lifetime.

Despite this vast spiritual awareness, remorse may remain in the heart. If left unprocessed, remorse becomes a heavy force that we bear emotionally and physically. According to the ancient traditions, unresolved emotions develop energetically in the body, eventually leading to illness or disease. Regrets, phobias, or unresolved emotions can all cause blockages in our energetic system, disturbing the normal flow of life force within us.

In this situation, energetic acceptance is critical. Accepting our life's decisions without judgement frees us from energetic links to the past. This discharge restores harmony to our system, eliminating energy stagnation, which can lead to illness. To age gracefully, we must free ourselves from the weight of regret, realising that holding on to previous mistakes simply drags us down, energetically and physically.

Forgiveness is an important part of letting go of regret – not just for others, but also for ourselves. We are generally tougher on ourselves than on others. We may harbour regrets about past relationships, professional decisions, or missed chances, believing that we could have done better. But forgiveness is the salve that enables us to heal. It is an admission that we did our best with the knowledge and resources available at the time.

Self-forgiveness releases the knots of regret in the heart and restores the free flow of energy throughout the body. This is more than just an emotional process; it is also energetic. When we forgive ourselves, we open clogged channels in our energetic body, allowing vitality to return to us. As a result, we promote our physical and emotional health, laying the groundwork for graceful ageing.

As we move through our years, it's important to cleanse ourselves of old energies that no longer serve our best interests. This cleansing process may occur on multiple levels, including emotional, mental, and energetic. Old regrets, unresolved emotions, and unhealed wounds are frequently brought to the surface in our older years – not as punishments, but as chances to heal. The body naturally slows down, allowing us more time to contemplate, process, and release.

This is when the wisdom of ageing really shines. With each passing year, we have the opportunity to let go of what no longer serves us. When we view our ageing process as a refinement of our energy, we open ourselves up to a tremendous transformation. We come to comprehend that every wrinkle and every grey hair, represents the lessons we've learned, the energy we've processed, and the peace we've achieved.

> This is when the wisdom of ageing really shines. With each passing year, we have the opportunity to let go of what no longer serves us.

At its foundation, energetic acceptance is about going with the natural flow of life. When we fight the current, whether through regret, resistance to ageing, or clinging to the past, we interrupt the natural flow of energy within us. However, when we submit and trust that our journey is unfolding as it should, we flow with the tide of life, allowing it to lead us smoothly towards our higher purpose.

This alignment is the key to ageing gracefully. It is not about conserving youth or rejecting the changes that occur throughout time. It is about accepting change as part of life's divine dance. When we release regrets, we free ourselves from the energetic loads of the past, allowing us to feel the lightness and clarity that comes with true acceptance.

Maintaining physical health, while vital, is not the only aspect of ageing successfully. It is about keeping energetic harmony – releasing what no longer serves us, forgiving ourselves for perceived mistakes, and accepting our chosen path without regret. In doing so, we allow ourselves to mature gracefully, wisely, and peacefully.

Energetic acceptance reminds us that life is not a sequence of right or wrong decisions, but rather a flowing river of experience, with each moment bringing us closer to our true nature. As we age, we are asked to embrace this flow, believing that we are always precisely where we are supposed to be, and that true well-being is found in our ability to accept and release with grace.

Casey Castro is the Founder of Primordial Path. Her work encompasses her experience in metaphysics, meditation, energy work, healings, esoteric practices, and psychology training.

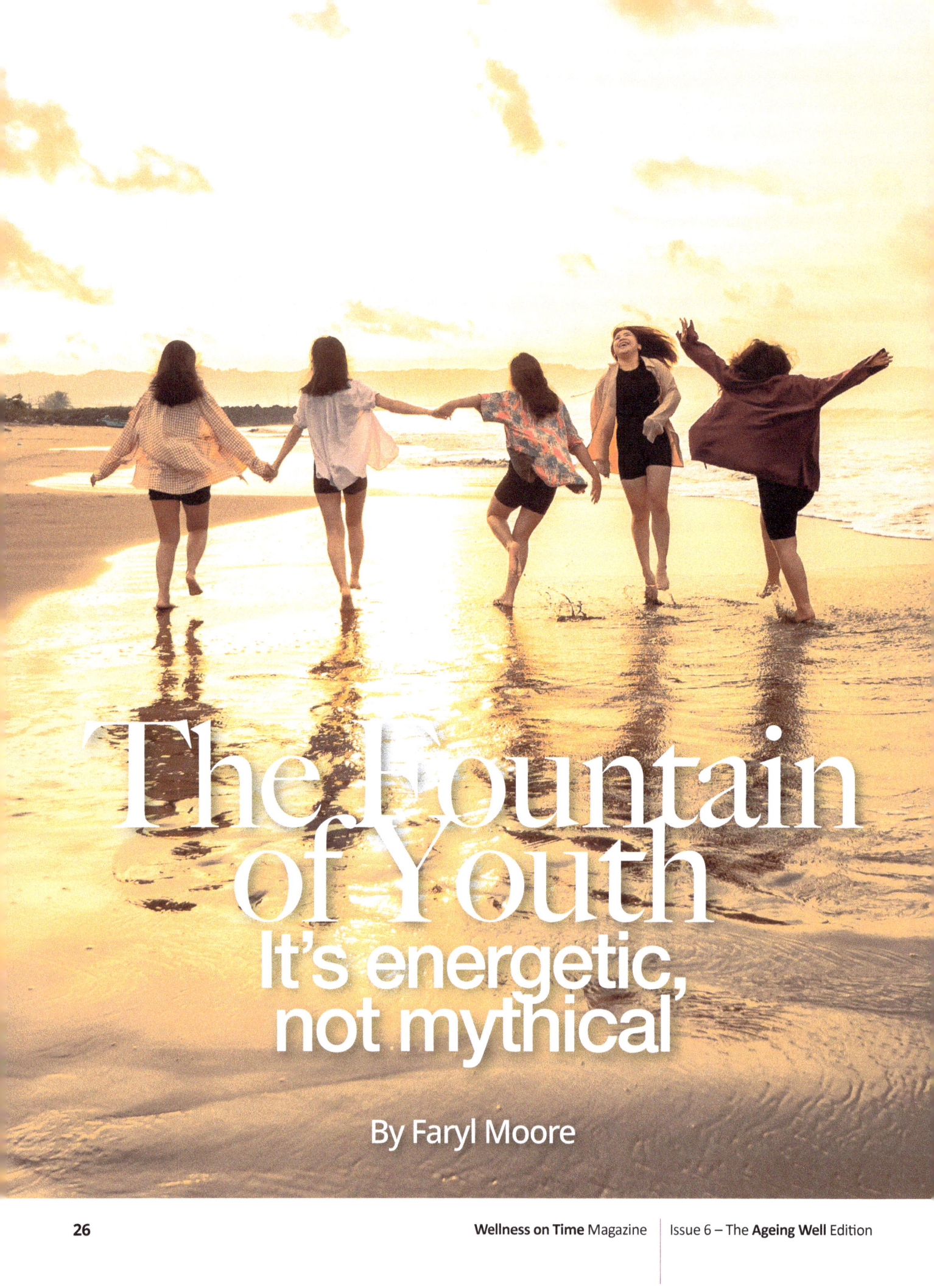

The Fountain of Youth

It's energetic, not mythical

By Faryl Moore

When we think of the Fountain of Youth, our minds often conjure images of magical waters that promise eternal youth to those who drink from them. But what if I told you that the real Fountain of Youth isn't something you need to search for in a far-off land? In fact, it's closer than you think. It's in your energy!

The energy-ageing connection

Let's get one thing straight – ageing isn't just about counting birthdays. It's about how your body, mind, and spirit hold up over time. And guess what? Your energy plays a starring role in this process. Stagnant or depleted energy is like a slow leak in a tyre. Over time, it can lead to physical and emotional imbalances, leaving you feeling worn out and, well, old.

In Pranic Healing, we see energy as the life force that animates your body and mind. When this energy flows freely and vibrantly, it nourishes every cell, organ, and thought. However, when your energy is blocked or depleted – whether from stress, poor habits, or unresolved emotions – it can contribute to the breakdown of your body's systems. Think of it as letting your inner garden wilt from neglect.

The real key to longevity

Longevity isn't about chasing the elusive ideal of perpetual youth. It's about embracing high vibes and letting your energy lead the way. Vibrant, flowing energy is like the best kind of anti-ageing cream, except it works from the inside out. It keeps you feeling youthful, not just looking it.

Maintaining vibrant energy requires conscious effort, but the rewards are well worth it. When your energy is high and balanced, you're not just surviving, you're thriving. Your body repairs itself more efficiently, your mind stays sharp, and your spirit remains light. It's like having a perpetual glow that no skincare routine can match. So here are some tips for cultivating the energy of longevity.

> **Keep your energy flowing:** regular energy practices like Pranic Healing, Yoga, or Tai Chi can help keep your energy pathways clear. It's like giving your energy system a regular tune-up to prevent stagnation.

> **Release what no longer serves you:** are you holding onto grudges, stress, or negative emotions? That's like carrying around emotional baggage that drains your energy. Let it go. You'll feel lighter, and your energy will thank you.

> **Nourish your body with high-vibe foods:** eating foods rich in prana – fresh fruits, vegetables, and whole grains – can boost your energy levels. Think of it as feeding your body the purest fuel available.

> **Surround yourself with positivity:** your environment and the people around you have a direct impact on your energy. Spend time in nature, cultivate positive relationships, and engage in activities that uplift you. High vibes attract more high vibes!

> **Stay connected to your purpose:** a strong sense of purpose is like an energy booster shot. When you're passionate about your life and what you're doing, your energy flows more freely, and you feel more vibrant.

> Surround yourself with positivity: your environment and the people around you have a direct impact on your energy. Spend time in nature, cultivate positive relationships, and engage in activities that uplift you. High vibes attract more high vibes!

In the end, longevity isn't about finding a mythical fountain or chasing youth – it's about embracing the power of your own energy. By keeping your energy vibrant and flowing, you can not only add years to your life, but life to your years. So, let your energy lead the way, and watch as you flourish with vitality, no matter your age.

Who knew the secret to a long, healthy life was so simple? Keep your vibes high and your energy flowing, and you might just find that the Fountain of Youth was within you all along.

Faryl Moore is a Professional Pranic Healer and Empowerment Coach, and Founder of Moore Energy.

If self-care, fun and joyous activities are important to you, schedule them in your diary first.

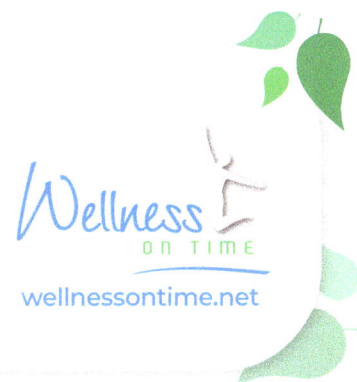

Wellness
on time
wellnessontime.net

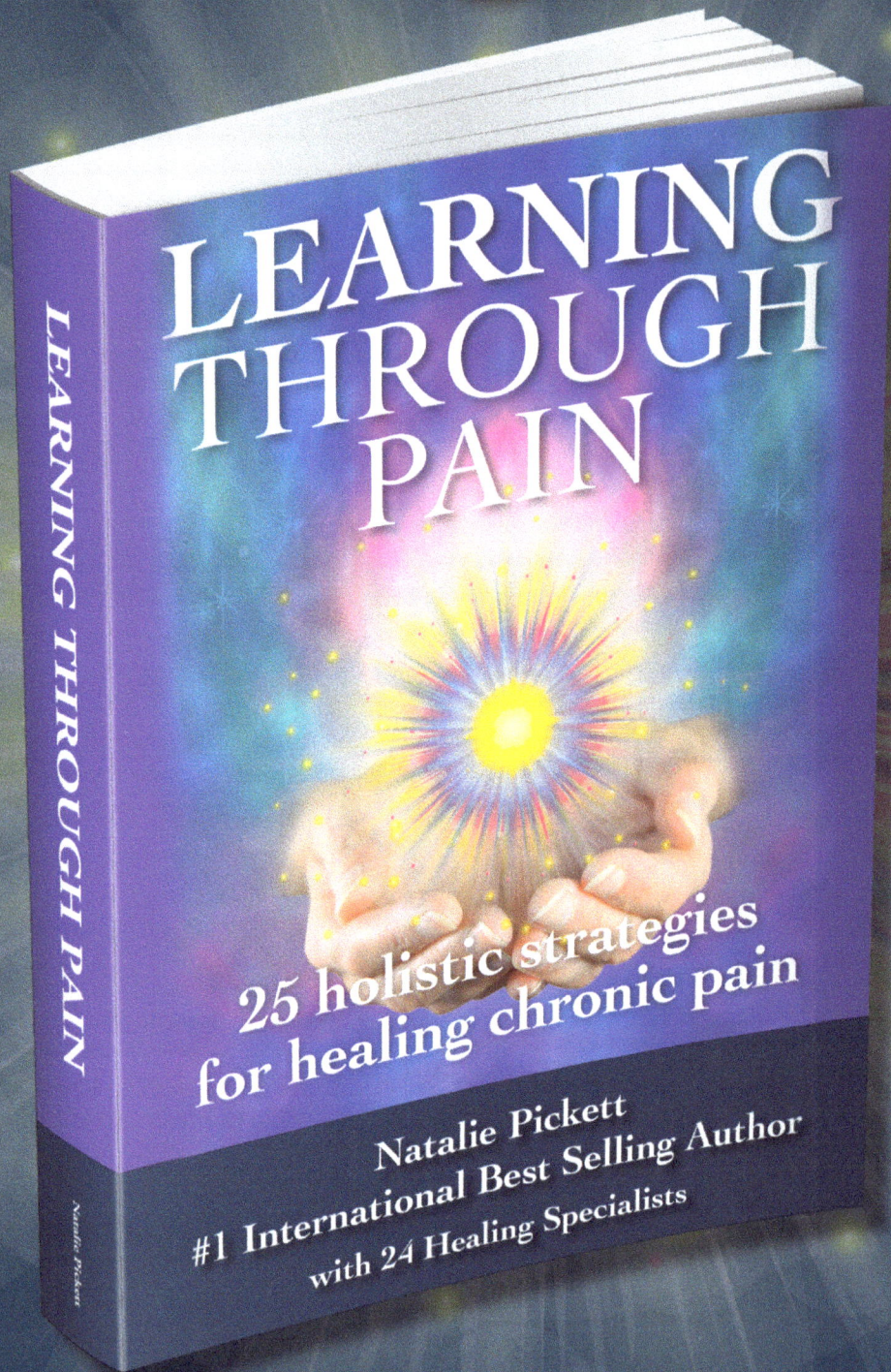

Ageing well

In this issue, we delve into the topic of ageing and how important ageing well is for our wellbeing.

For most of us as we get older, one of the things we notice is that we don't 'bounce back' quite like we used to! There may be times when our energy feels low, not what it once was. In recent years, rather than see this as a loss, I've come to understand this as an opportunity to connect more with my body and be in tune to what it needs.

Our energy is more than just our physical energy, it is also the intangible energy field that we cannot see but can definitely feel. Our energy is an incredibly valuable resource, and if we constantly give, eventually it will deplete, and the pattern of giving more than we get back will eventually take its toll.

As an entrepreneur for 30 years with multiple businesses, as well as a mum, I've had my share of life experience. There is the constant juggle to prioritise business or family, and it's easy to fall into the habit of spending a lot of your day doing activities that drain your energy. I know from past experience how important it is to take time to restore your energy, because by the time we've reached burnout, it has probably taken years of neglecting our needs.

My big 'Aha!' moment was when I realised I didn't need to say 'Yes!' to everything. I began to be selective about the clients, projects and activities I engaged with. Taking time to slow down, not rush, do a little bit at a time, and remove stress from my daily routine guided me to the discovery that there's plenty of time, and everything still gets done. Today, I value being able to work to my own pace and not be influenced by other people's agendas.

I'm happiest when I am doing things that restore my energy, and sometimes that is working on projects that feed my soul, or simply taking time out. If there is something that you want to do but you haven't been making the time for it, the starting point is for you to make it a priority. Put it in your diary and don't move it for anything else. This is the richness of life, and it is another definition of 'success' that I value – when I make time in my day to do things that bring me joy.

Changing the habit to prioritise yourself does take some reminding. I don't always get this right, but I have reset my focus to listening to my body and how I am feeling. I resist the need to 'push through' and take heed when my body and spirit are telling me to take a break.

It is encouraging to see more awareness of how important wellness is to our lives. As human beings, it is all intertwined – how we feel emotionally and mentally relates to how we feel physically.

It is said that life is about the journey, and evolving to be more in tune with how we feel is important. Perhaps that's the wisdom that comes with ageing. For me, this is about continuous growth and learning to create my best life. Making sure that I honour my connection with all elements of myself – mind, body, soul, heart, and spirit – is key to my life balance.

It's a common thread. These shared lived experiences of seeking answers or discovering solutions inspires and empowers people to become advocates, share their knowledge, provide support, and sometimes pivot their careers to wellness. Everyone's pathway in life is different, and it is important to be open to try new things.

As a best-selling author, my enthusiasm for sharing discoveries that work led me to create this magazine as well as the soon-to-be-released book *Learning Through Pain*, where 25 authors share their ideas and strategies to help improve wellbeing.

Searching the globe for contributors from a range of practices who have a common goal to share their wellness knowledge and experience, has brought together this interview series. By sharing their stories, they are making a difference in their own lives and the lives of others. It is an honour to share these 'Ageing Well' interviews with Prema Joy and Laura Gindac who discovered the importance of wellness in their lives, sought to find answers, and wanted to share their knowledge to help others.

Thank you for trusting us with your stories and allowing us to share them with the world.

— **Natalie Pickett, Wellness on Time CEO, Founder, Publisher, Editor-in-Chief**

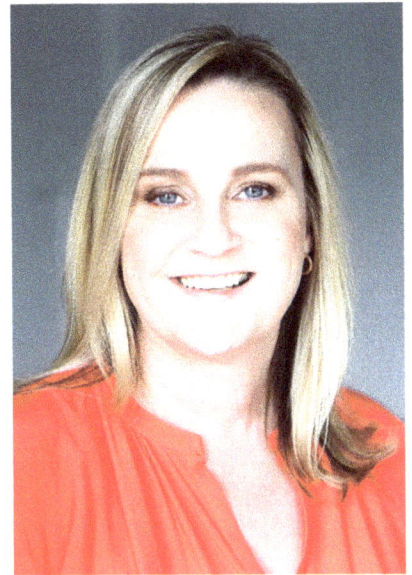

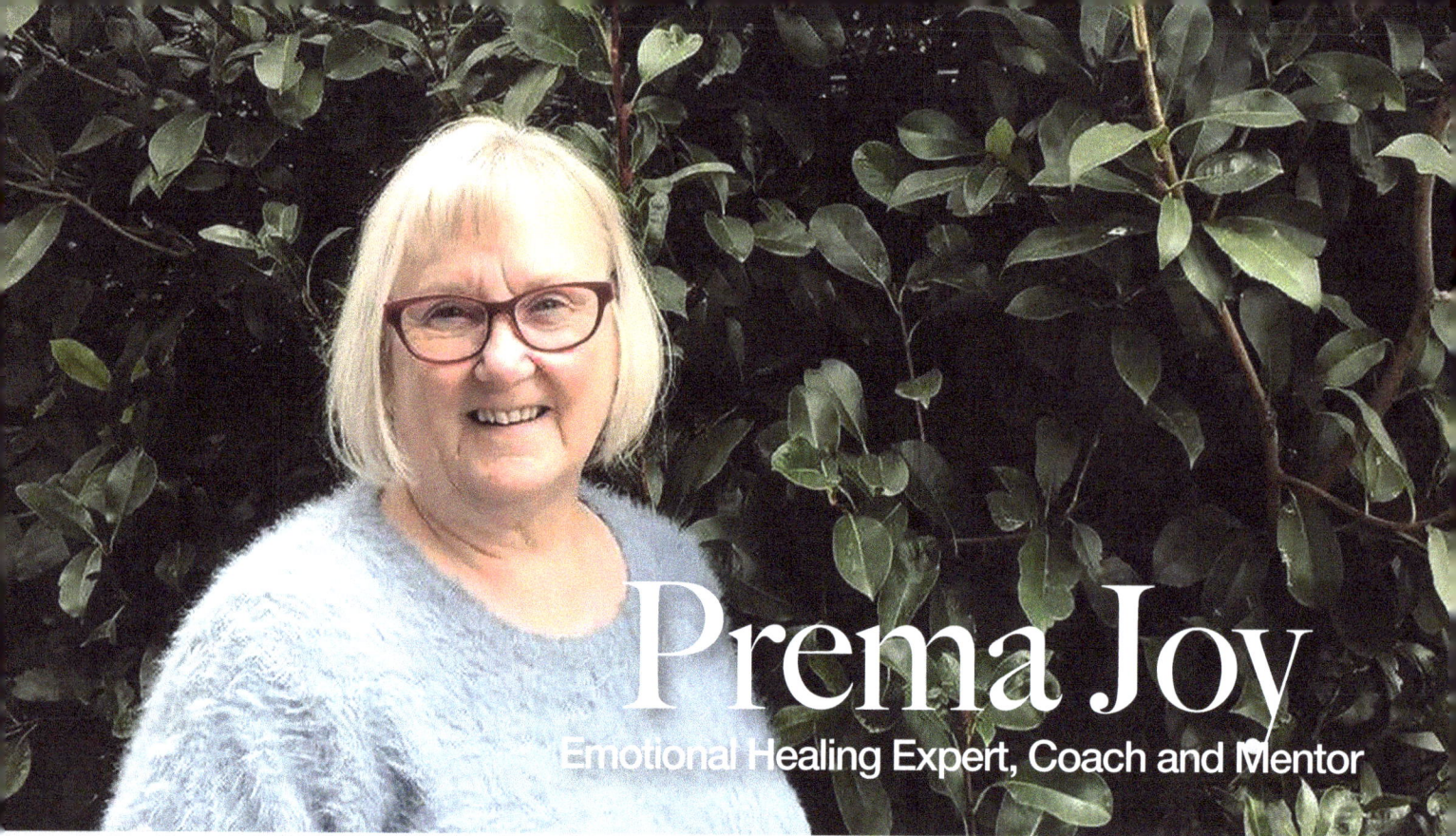

Prema Joy

Emotional Healing Expert, Coach and Mentor

Please tell us about the work that you do as a practitioner or advocate in the wellness industry?

I am in Adelaide, South Australia. I am an Emotional Healing Expert, Author, Speaker, Journey Practitioner, Coach and Mentor with three decades of self-development experience. I am a lover of truth, self-love, vibrant health, endless cups of tea, dogs, travel, belly laughs, nature, my grandies/family, singing, dancing, drumming, ice-cream, painting, sunsets, and life – however it shows up.

Have you always had an interest in wellness?

My journey of wellness began 32 years ago when I walked away from domestic violence and alcoholism. Healing my self-worth issues and addictions led me to gain many insights and skills. At age 12, I'd found my father dead, and a few short months later we left England for Australia. I held unexpressed grief for my dad, home, dog, friends, and school for 30 years.

Healing myself emotionally became a passion and has led to helping and inspiring others to open, delve into their own healing, find forgiveness, and accept happiness and wellness in their lives.

> Healing myself emotionally ... has led to helping and inspiring others to open, delve into their own healing, find forgiveness, and accept happiness and wellness in their lives.

After a profound trip to India in 2015 where a Master gave me the spiritual name Prema, I decided to keep it and change my name. My middle name had always been Joy, so I became Prema Joy.

What are your thoughts around the topic of ageing well, and how can our readers use this for their benefit?

I believe to truly age well, our mind, physical body and emotional body need harmony, and that wellness comes from within. When you love and trust yourself, you become aware of your thoughts, tune in to the messages from your body, and open the heart/soul purpose and expression. Your self-nurturing grows, your body energy systems replenish, and you end up naturally open in a pre-dispositioned place of wellness and connection.

> When you love and trust yourself, you become aware of your thoughts, tune in to the messages from your body, and open the heart/soul purpose and expression.

Can you remember when you first realised the importance of wellness in your daily life? Was there an 'Aha!' moment like you'd solved a life puzzle? What was the impetus to start doing what you do as a career choice?

In 2005 at my first Journey Intensive, I got a direct experience of my own Source – to know myself as everything and that everything was love. It changed everything in me. For the first time in my life, I knew the truth of who I was, and am, and that truth began to unfold exponentially in my life.

This 'Aha!' moment gave me permission to allow my emotions to flow freely, healthily, and then I began to take responsibility for my own actions. I stopped blaming outside influences, circumstances, my past, and other people. I stopped running and hiding from myself. I forgave myself and others, and realised that it was my choice to abuse or approve of myself, and that I had the power to choose wellness.

A passion was born in me to serve others – to help them discover for themselves their own truth.

How long did it take for you to start working with this area of wellness? Did you do any special training and try a few different things before you found the right healing modalities for you?

After leaving my ex-husband in 1994, I became an astrologer, past-life therapist, clairvoyant tarot reader, and energy healer. It wasn't until I did the training as a Journey Practitioner that I truly began deeply healing, and the path to wellness and my work flourished.

Can you provide a top tip for our readers on how to manage and integrate wellness activities into their day?

Get into your body! The body never lies, and the mind is always full of stories. Integrate one thing daily; deep breaths before you get out of bed, meditation, walk in nature, grass, beach, hug a tree, drum, sing, dance, yoga, move, paint ... because any of these will get you back into your body. When you're in your body, your mind will quieten, relax, and stress less.

> Get into your body! The body never lies, and the mind is always full of stories. Integrate one thing daily; deep breaths before you get out of bed, meditation, walk in nature, grass, beach, hug a tree, drum, sing, dance, yoga, move, paint ... because any of these will get you back into your body.

In you could describe the importance of ageing well for our readers in three words, what would they be?

Fully expressed life.

Explore ...

🌐 www.premajoy.com

f https://www.facebook.com/profile.php?id=100075648859161

f https://www.facebook.com/profile.php?id=100063662135619

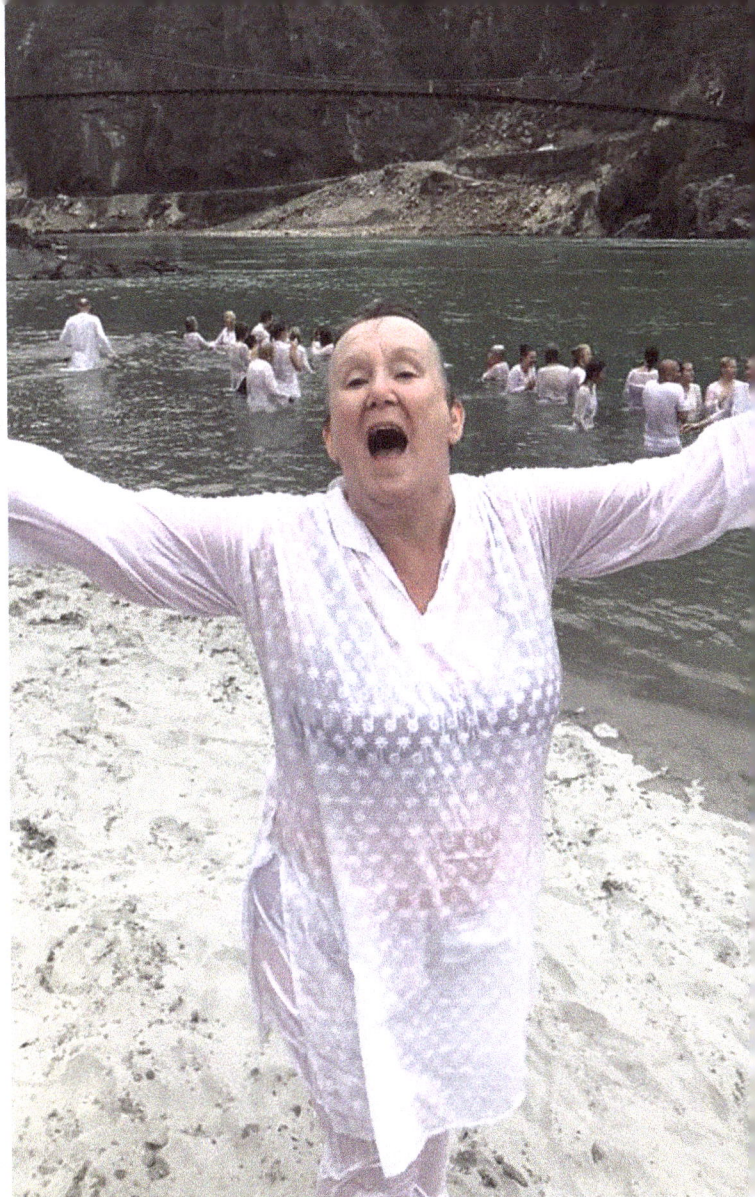

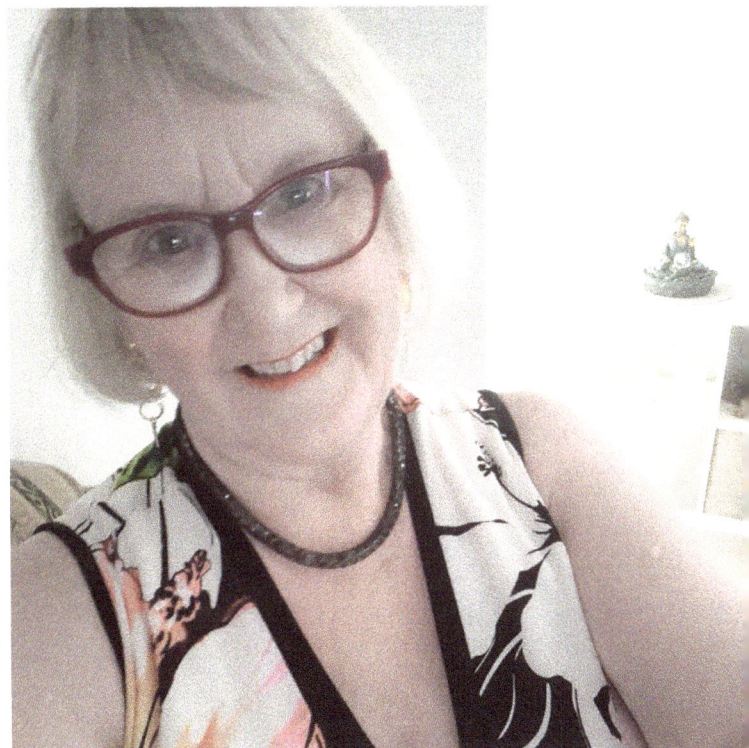

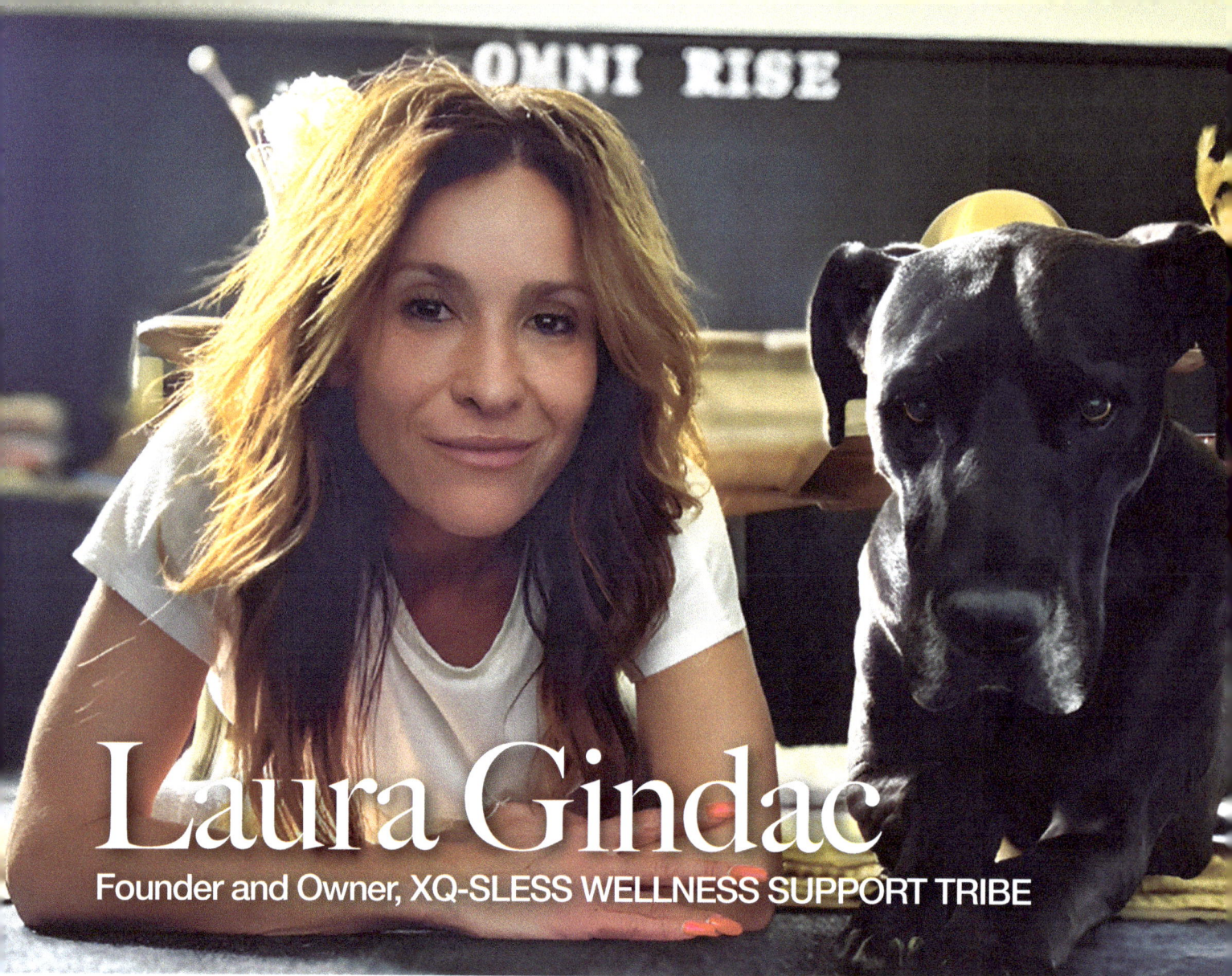

Laura Gindac

Founder and Owner, XQ-SLESS WELLNESS SUPPORT TRIBE

Please tell us a bit about the work that you do as a practitioner or advocate in the wellness industry.

After nearly 20 years in the high-pressure, male-dominated automotive industry, I realised the need for a shift. While excelling in fast-paced corporate environments, I understood the importance of balance and well-being. I decided to take the bold step to leave behind the familiar and embark on my own journey of self-discovery and entrepreneurship.

> While excelling in fast-paced corporate environments, I understood the importance of balance and well-being.

I now channel my deep expertise in high-achieving sales strategies and leadership to create a structured curriculum for those committed to personal and professional growth. My vision combines high-level business strategies with transformative wellness principles, driven by my dedication to yoga and meditation.

As the Australian ambassador for Pursuit 365, I select entrepreneurs from around the world to share their stories, fuelling a new generation of visionary leaders. My passion is clear – to shape the future of business by blending excellence with well-being.

Have you always had an interest in wellness?

At 10, my world shattered with a single tragic event. Fear took root, and my once-safe home felt like a place of danger. As I grew into my teens, I realised everything around me felt distant and unreal. Anxiety became my constant companion, though no one had a name for it back then. My family sought help from countless doctors, but no one could explain what was happening to me.

In my 20s, I turned to self-help books, grateful they became my refuge instead of the drugs and alcohol that surrounded me. Yet, despite all the reading, I was still lost in confusion. It wasn't until I found joy in dancing that I felt a brief release from the storm inside my mind. But it wasn't until my late 30s that I stumbled upon the concept of the nervous system. That's when it all clicked – I'd been living in 'fight or flight' mode for most of my life. And my journey to wellness finally began.

What are your thoughts around the topic of ageing well, and how can our readers use this for their benefit?

'Ageing well' is simply a term to describe the unfolding of thinking and feeling well. Many believe that ageing well is connected to what the beauty industry calls 'beauty'. However, this term is a superficial fabrication based on an influential, biased opinion that dictates what beauty is. If something is delightful to the senses, we call it 'beautiful'. The only true beauty is in the delight of being well.

> If something is delightful to the senses, we call it 'beautiful'. The only true beauty is in the delight of being well.

Can you remember when you first realised the importance of wellness in your daily life? Was there an 'Aha!' moment like you'd solved a life puzzle? What was the impetus to start doing what you do as a career choice.

I realised that if I wanted a life of true wellness, it had to be woven into my everyday routine. And what better way to do that than by making it part of my work? I knew that what we focus on each day shapes our lives, so I started planting seeds of wellness everywhere I could – nurturing myself while helping others along the way. That's when Omni-Rise was born, from a deep desire to grow and uplift within myself and in the lives of those around me.

How long did it take for you to start working with this area of wellness? Did you do any special training and try a few different things before you found the right healing modalities for you?

I immersed myself in learning everything I could about the human mind, brain, and body, studying day and night. I explored modern science and esoteric knowledge, seeking answers from every possible angle. Through all this, one truth became clear – a calm mind can take care of everything else. It's a paradox, really ... how something as simple as meditation, just being still and doing nothing, can produce massive results that no amount of physical effort ever could.

Can you provide a top tip for our readers on how to manage and integrate wellness activities into their day?

Carve out a few minutes each day to be still, to think well, to move well, to eat well, and to give.

In you could describe the importance of ageing well for our readers in three words, what would they be?

Firstly, honour yourself.

Is there anything further you would like to add?

Wherever you find yourself in life is the dawn of a new journey. Every moment is a fresh canvas, inviting you to begin anew. Start your count from this very instant. Numbers are mere tools, shaped by the dreams we weave and the stories we craft; they represent nothing more than the essence of our creations.

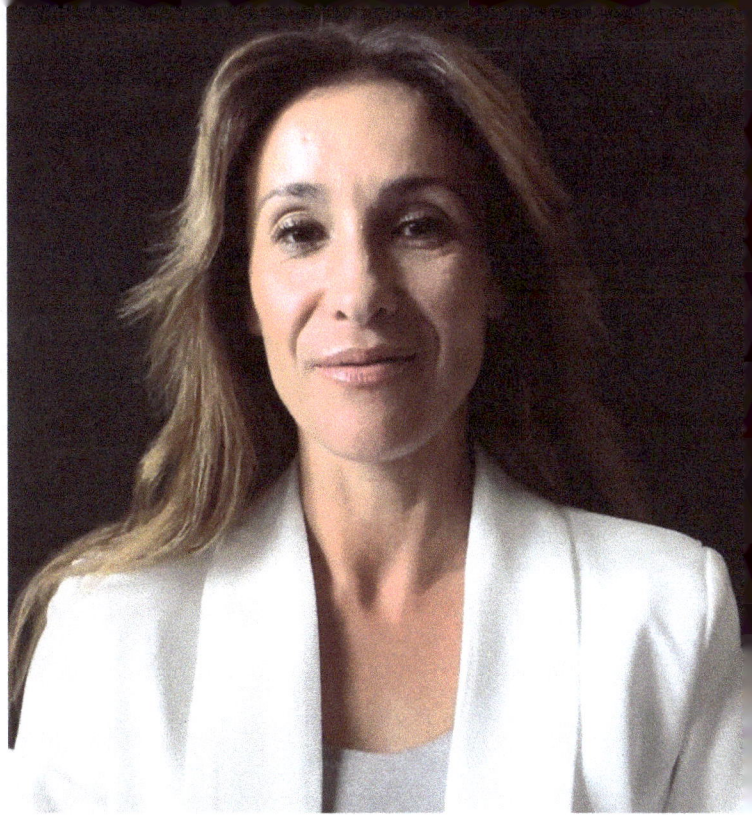

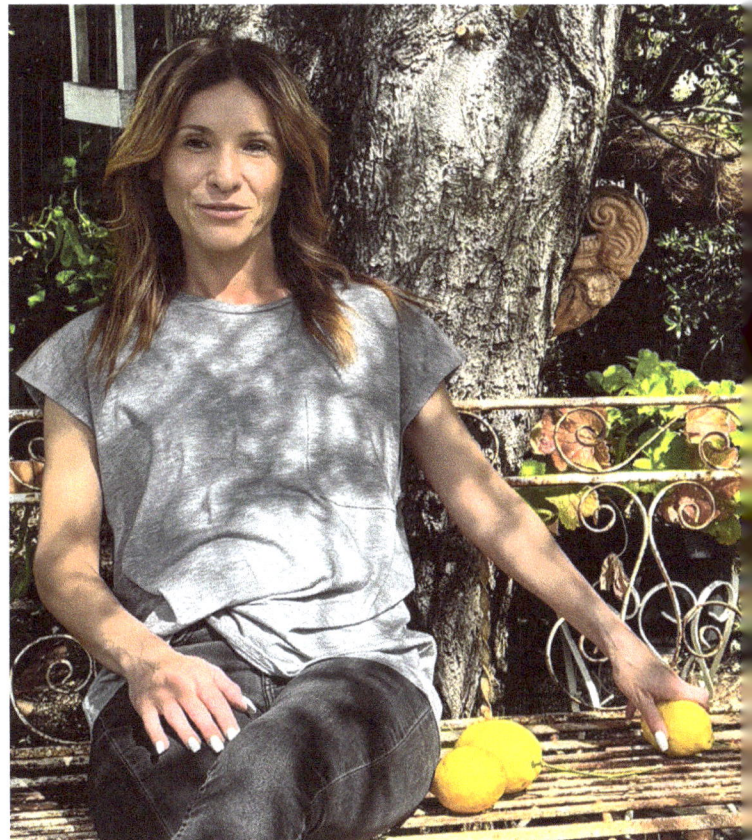

Explore ...

🌐 www.omnirisetraining.com

📘 https://www.facebook.com/profile.php?id=100033892417334

📷 https://www.instagram.com/omni_rise_training_/

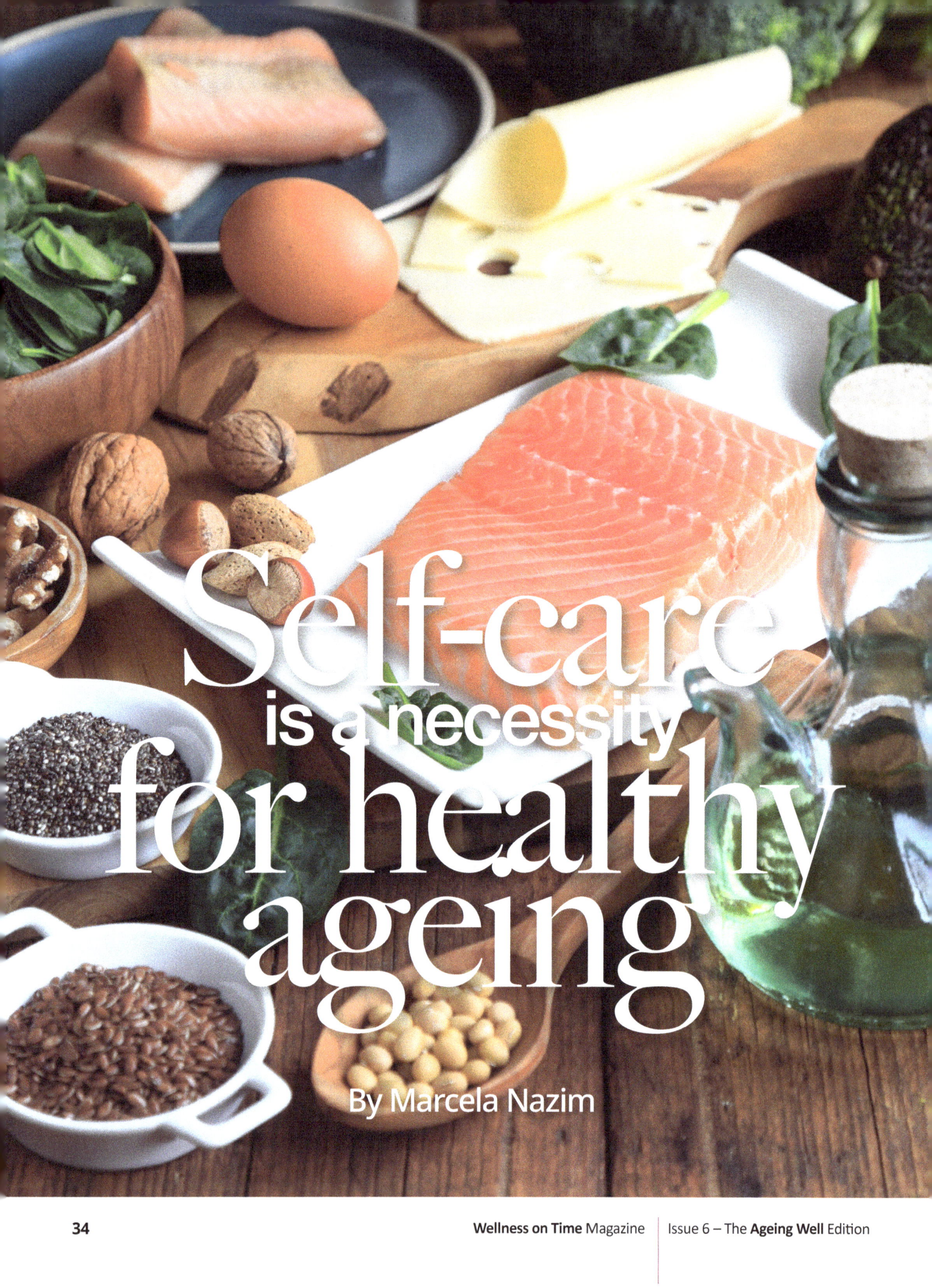

Self-care is a necessity for healthy ageing

By Marcela Nazim

> '**S**o many women I've talked to see this time as an ending. But I have discovered that this is your time to reinvent yourself after years of focusing on the needs of everyone else.'
> — Oprah Winfrey

When posed with the question of what they sacrifice the most, a resounding truth emerges – self-care and prioritising personal well-being often take a backseat for many women. The endless juggling act of responsibilities – be it advancing careers or tending to family needs – can leave us feeling depleted and running on empty.

Amidst this chaos, it's all too easy to place yourself last on your list of priorities. Like many women, I once believed that a new face cream or the latest supplement was enough self-care. It took minimal effort, and after all, I had so much to do for everyone else. But I've since learned that true self-care goes far deeper. It demands more than the occasional spa day; it requires a holistic approach to ensure healthy ageing and hormonal balance. As Dr Mindy Peltz (Author of *The Menopause Reset*) writes, 'Self-care isn't a luxury; it's a necessity for hormonal balance.'

The role of hormones during perimenopause

This time marks significant hormonal fluctuations in a woman's body as it prepares for menopause. For some women, the time leading up to the big event called perimenopause, which Gail Sheehy (Author of *The Wisdom of Menopause*) refers to as '... a second Spring when every woman can become who she was meant to be', can take up to 10 years. During this period, our hormone levels – especially estrogen, progesterone, and testosterone – fluctuate significantly, leading to a host of physical and emotional symptoms.

Estrogen: this primary female hormone begins to decrease during perimenopause. Lower estrogen levels can cause irregular periods, hot flashes, and night sweats. It also affects mood, memory, and bone health.

Progesterone: as estrogen levels decline, progesterone levels drop too, leading to irregular periods and sleep disturbances. Progesterone also helps regulate mood, so its decrease can contribute to feelings of anxiety or depression.

Testosterone: often associated with men, testosterone is also crucial for women's libido, energy levels, and muscle mass. Declining testosterone can lead to fatigue, reduced sex drive, and difficulty maintaining muscle tone.

The necessity of self-care for hormonal balance

Understanding these hormonal changes underlines the importance of self-care during perimenopause. It's not a luxury or something to fit in when we have time; it's a necessity. Here are some suggestions on how we can balance our hormones and overall well-being holistically.

1. Nutrition: feed your hormones

A diet rich in whole foods – fruits, vegetables, lean proteins, and healthy fats – provides the nutrients our body needs to produce and regulate hormones. Incorporating foods high in omega-3 fatty acids, like salmon and flaxseeds, can help reduce inflammation and support brain health. Phytoestrogens – found in foods like soy, flaxseeds, and chickpeas – can mimic estrogen and help balance hormones naturally.

> A diet rich in whole foods ... provides the nutrients our body needs to produce and regulate hormones. Incorporating foods high in omega-3 fatty acids, like salmon and flaxseeds, can help reduce inflammation and support brain health.

2. Exercise: keep moving

Regular physical activity helps regulate insulin, boost metabolism, and reduce stress, all of which are crucial during perimenopause. A combination of cardio and strength training supports heart health and maintain muscle mass. Exercise also promotes the release of endorphins, improving mood and combating perimenopausal symptoms like anxiety and depression.

3. Sleep: prioritise rest

Quality sleep is essential for hormone production and overall health. Establish a regular sleep routine, create a calming bedtime environment, and limiting caffeine and screen time before bed helps improve sleep quality.

4. Stress management: balance cortisol

Chronic stress leads to elevated cortisol levels, which can worsen hormonal imbalances. Incorporate stress relief techniques like meditation, yoga, or deep breathing into your daily routine to keep cortisol in check.

Don't suffer in silence

Finally, remember that we don't have to navigate perimenopause alone. Talk to your friends, share your experiences, and seek medical advice if needed. Hormonal changes can feel overwhelming, but with the right self-care strategies, we don't have to settle for just feeling okay – we deserve to, and can, feel great! Investing in ourselves isn't just about looking good on the outside; it's about nurturing our body from within. As we age, investing in self-care is the key to not just surviving but thriving.

Marcela Nazim is a Health Coach, Yoga Instructor, Sport and Weight Loss Nutritionist, as well as a Wife and a Mother.

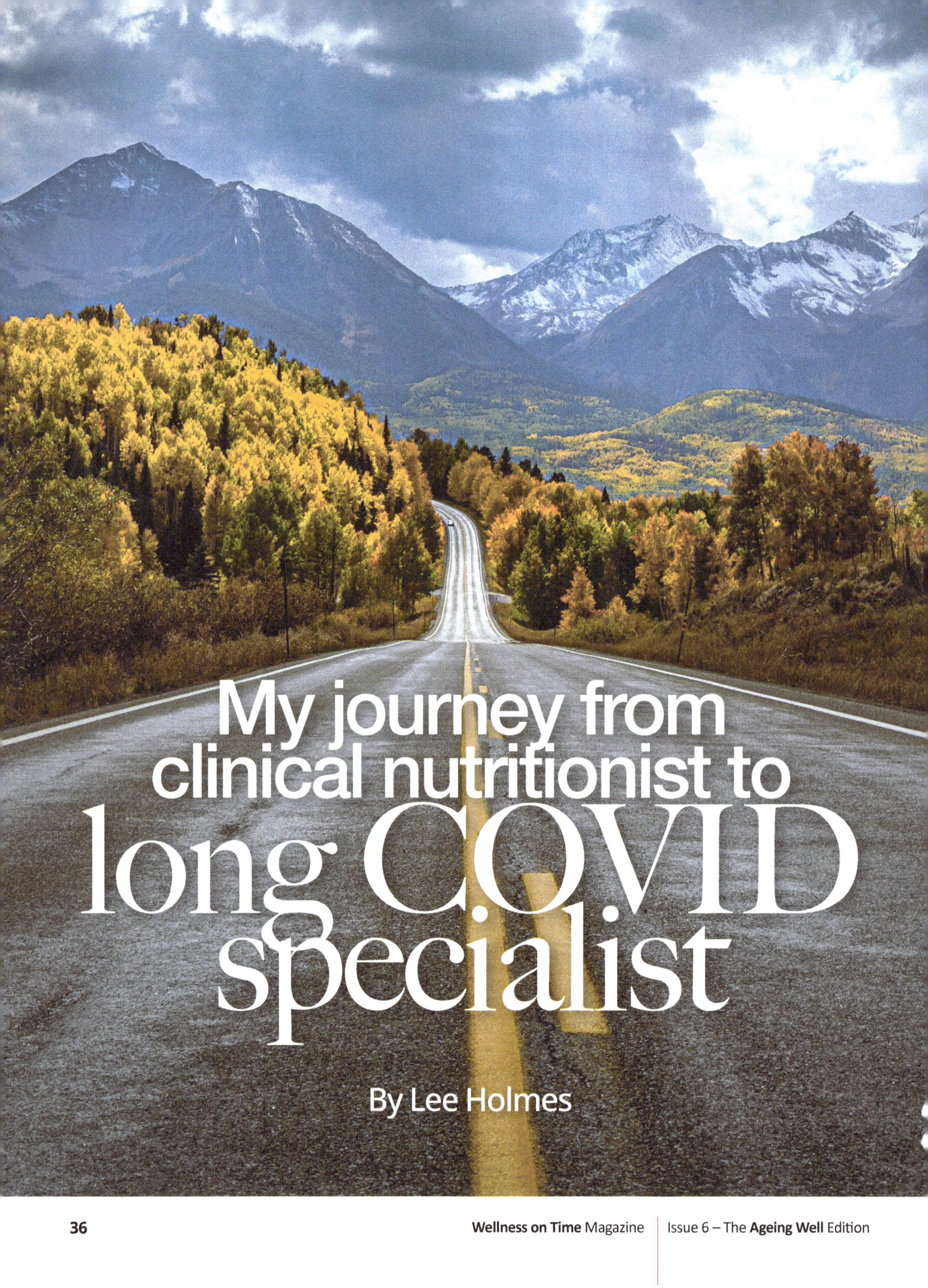

My journey from clinical nutritionist to long COVID specialist

By Lee Holmes

As a clinical nutritionist and bestselling author of ten books on health and nutrition, I never anticipated becoming intimately acquainted with long COVID. Yet, in April 2022 during a trip to England, I contracted COVID-19, setting me on an unexpected journey that would profoundly reshape my understanding of health and wellness.

This experience has not only challenged me personally, but also fuelled my passion for exploring emerging trends in long COVID treatment and management. Finding myself unexpectedly on the patient's side of healthcare, I've been driven to delve deeper into the complexities of this condition, exploring current research, and innovative treatment approaches.

Through my research and personal experience, I've uncovered emerging trends and strategies that offer new hope to those affected by long COVID. In this article, I aim to guide you through these cutting-edge developments – from novel dietary approaches to ground-breaking medical treatments – and share insights into how the medical community's understanding of long COVID is evolving and being adapted within its approach to care.

Whether you're living with long COVID yourself, supporting someone who is, or seeking to understand this condition better, my goal is to provide you with valuable, up-to-date information that can make a tangible difference. Looking at the most recent advancements in long COVID management, here are my most used treatment and management tools that I use in my clinic to create an individualised roadmap.

1. Understanding the role of mast cells and histamine

Recent research has illuminated the significant role that mast cells and histamine play in perpetuating long COVID symptoms. Mast cells, integral to allergic reactions and inflammation, can become hyperactive in individuals with long COVID, leading to chronic inflammation and a spectrum of symptoms. Adopting a low-histamine diet can help manage these symptoms by reducing the body's histamine load. This approach emphasises the importance of low-histamine fresh fruits and vegetables, proteins, and gluten-free grains.

2. Personalised nutrition plans

Nutrition has emerged as a cornerstone in managing long COVID. Personalised nutrition plans focusing on anti-inflammatory foods, gut health, and nutrient optimisation are key. These plans and the protocol I use in my book *Nature's Way to Healing. A Long COVID Guide*, emphasises foods rich in omega-3 fatty acids, antioxidants, and probiotics, tailored to individual needs to manage symptoms and support overall recovery. Supplements such as vitamin D, vitamin C, and zinc are frequently incorporated.

3. Rest and pacing strategies

The critical importance of rest and pacing in long COVID management cannot be overstated. Post-exertional malaise (PEM), where symptoms worsen after physical or mental exertion, is a common challenge. Learning to listen to one's body, incorporating frequent rest periods, and utilising tools like activity diaries and pacing apps are crucial strategies for managing energy levels and preventing symptom flare-ups.

4. Mind-body therapies

Integrating mind-body therapies such as yoga, meditation, and breathing exercises has shown promise in regulating the nervous system and reducing stress for long COVID patients. These practices promote relaxation, improve mental clarity, and enhance overall well-being. Techniques like progressive muscle relaxation and mindfulness meditation are particularly beneficial in managing the mental and emotional strain of long COVID.

5. Holistic and integrative approaches

A multifaceted approach to treatment is essential for managing the diverse and complex symptoms of long COVID. Combining conventional medical treatments with complementary therapies, such as acupuncture and herbal supplements, allows for a more comprehensive and individualised care plan. Nutritional options like quercetin, ginger, and turmeric are being explored for their potential benefits in managing symptoms.

6. Physical rehabilitation and exercise therapy

Gradual and supervised physical rehabilitation programs are proving beneficial for long COVID patients. These programs focus on rebuilding strength and stamina without triggering PEM. Techniques such as graded exercise therapy (GET) and pacing are employed to help patients gradually increase their activity levels. Physiotherapy, tailored to individual tolerance and progress, is a critical component of recovery.

Long COVID has taught me that health is not a destination but a journey. It has reinforced the importance of compassion – for others and ourselves. As I continue to heal and help others, I carry a deeper understanding of the often-invisible battles many of us face, and what it means to be truly healthy.

This experience has transformed me – not just as a health practitioner, but as a person. It has reinforced my commitment to holistic health and provided a new perspective on the intricate connections between our bodies, minds, and the world around us. Through this challenging journey, I've found a renewed purpose – to be a voice for those struggling with long COVID, and to continue exploring innovative ways to support healing and wellness in all its forms.

Lee Holmes is an Accredited Clinical Nutritionist, Founder of Supercharged Foods, and Best-Selling Author of ten books including *Nature's Way to Healing: A Long COVID Guide*.

Medical Qi Gong
Reclaiming the life force as our birthright

By Deepa Gleason

Medical Qi Gong is a powerful and ancient practice within Traditional Chinese Medicine (TCM) that emphasises the cultivation, movement, and transformation of 'Qi', or life force energy. 'Qi' (pronounced 'Chee') refers to the vital energy that flows through all living beings, and 'Gong' means skill. Thus, Qi Gong can be understood as the art of mastering one's life force energy. Through this mastery, we can improve our health, well-being, and overall vitality. In this way, Qi Gong is akin to other energy-based healing systems, such as acupuncture, yoga, reiki, and even certain forms of breathwork and massage, all of which aim to move, augment, or redirect the life force.

In ancient Chinese traditions, it was understood that all illness – physical and emotional – stems from imbalances in the flow of Qi. Whether it is an excess, deficiency, or stagnation of energy, these imbalances disrupt the body's natural harmony and lead to the sensation of being unwell and disease. The concept of life force energy as a determinant of health is also central to many traditional healing systems across the world – from the chakra-based energy management system in Vedic healing to the Prana in yoga. Sadly, modern society has lost its connection to this knowledge, discarding the innate sensitivity to energy that is our birthright in favor of relinquishing autonomy to external authorities.

As women, especially as we age and enter the crone or wise woman stage of life, this sensitivity to energy often resurfaces. You may have noticed that with age, you begin to sense energy more intuitively. Perhaps you think of a friend, and they call or text you shortly after, or you instinctively know when a family member is struggling. This isn't merely coincidence – it is the manifestation of energy at work. Women, particularly in the later stages of life, have cultivated an innate ability to read and sense energy through years of living, feeling, and connecting. This wisdom and sensitivity have always been within us, but we are often taught to ignore or suppress it in favour of rational, external sources of knowledge. Now is the time to reclaim and recognise that there is more to life that what we see.

Energy is the foundation of all matter, and movement in energy precedes movement in the physical world. Einstein's famous equation – $E=MC^2$ – demonstrates this scientifically; energy and matter are interchangeable, two expressions of the same substance. This concept is at the core of medical Qi Gong and other energy healing traditions. Before a physical illness can manifest in the body, there is always an energetic imbalance. By addressing the energy – through breath, movement, visualisation, or prayer – healing can take place on a fundamental level before the physical symptoms arise.

This understanding has even found its way into modern Western medicine, though perhaps in more subtle forms. Tests such as electroencephalograms (EEGs) (measuring brain activity), electrocardiograms (ECGs or EKGs) (measuring heart activity), and electromyographys (EMGs) (measuring muscle response), all document the movement of energy in the body in waveforms. While Western medicine often focuses on the physical symptoms that result from energy imbalances, traditional systems like medical Qi Gong recognise that resolving the energetic disturbance itself can prevent or heal the illness entirely. The rivers of energy that flow through our bodies, known as Meridians in TCM, and Nadis in Ayurveda, must move freely in their proper channels. If blocked or misdirected, these energy pathways create dysfunction, pain, and disease. This is why practices like acupuncture, herbal treatments, and Qi Gong itself are used to restore balance and promote the free flow of Qi.

The wisdom of these ancient systems goes back thousands of years, with traditional Chinese energy healing practices recorded on tortoise shells long before they discovered paper. These treatments are still in use today, proving their enduring efficacy. Compare this to the relatively recent discovery of antibiotics, like penicillin, which are less than 100 years old. While modern medicine has its place, we must not lose sight of the fact that the manipulation of energy – whether through intention, breathwork, visualisation, herbs, or movement – has been healing humanity for millennia.

> While modern medicine has its place, we must not lose sight of the fact that the manipulation of energy – whether through intention, breathwork, visualisation, herbs, or movement – has been healing humanity for millennia.

For women entering the crone stage, there is a natural reconnection to this energy work. As we age, our sensitivity to the subtle flows of Qi often intensifies. The crone is a symbol of wisdom, maturity, and deepened connection to life's mysteries. We begin to perceive the world energetically – whether through the shimmering 'sparkles' of intuitive insight, or the ability to sense and manipulate energy in ourselves and others. This awareness is a gift, a birthright that has been honed over a lifetime of experiences. Far from being something to fear, ageing offers us the opportunity to embrace our role as healers, teachers, and wise women, connected to the life force that flows through all things. We are gifted the opportunity to share this wisdom with those around us, and that is the best legacy one can leave. Knowledge of self-care and healing on a most profound level.

Science, too, has begun to acknowledge the profound reality of energy. In modern physics, subatomic particles are not only classified by their mass but also by their energy states, with properties like 'spin' and 'colour' used to describe them. These terms reflect the inherent vibrational and energetic nature of the Universe, further validating what traditional healers have known for thousands of years.

Medical Qi Gong offers a pathway to health by addressing the fundamental forces of life itself. By embracing the flow of life force energy, we not only improve our health but also reconnect with the deeper wisdom that is our birthright. This journey of energy mastery is ancient and modern, scientific and spiritual, and above all, it is a reminder that the power to heal lies within us all.

Deepa Gleason RN is an Acupuncturist, Healer and Teacher of Healing Arts based in Costa Rica, on her 200-acre nature reserve and organic farm called Granja Integral Luz del Corazon.

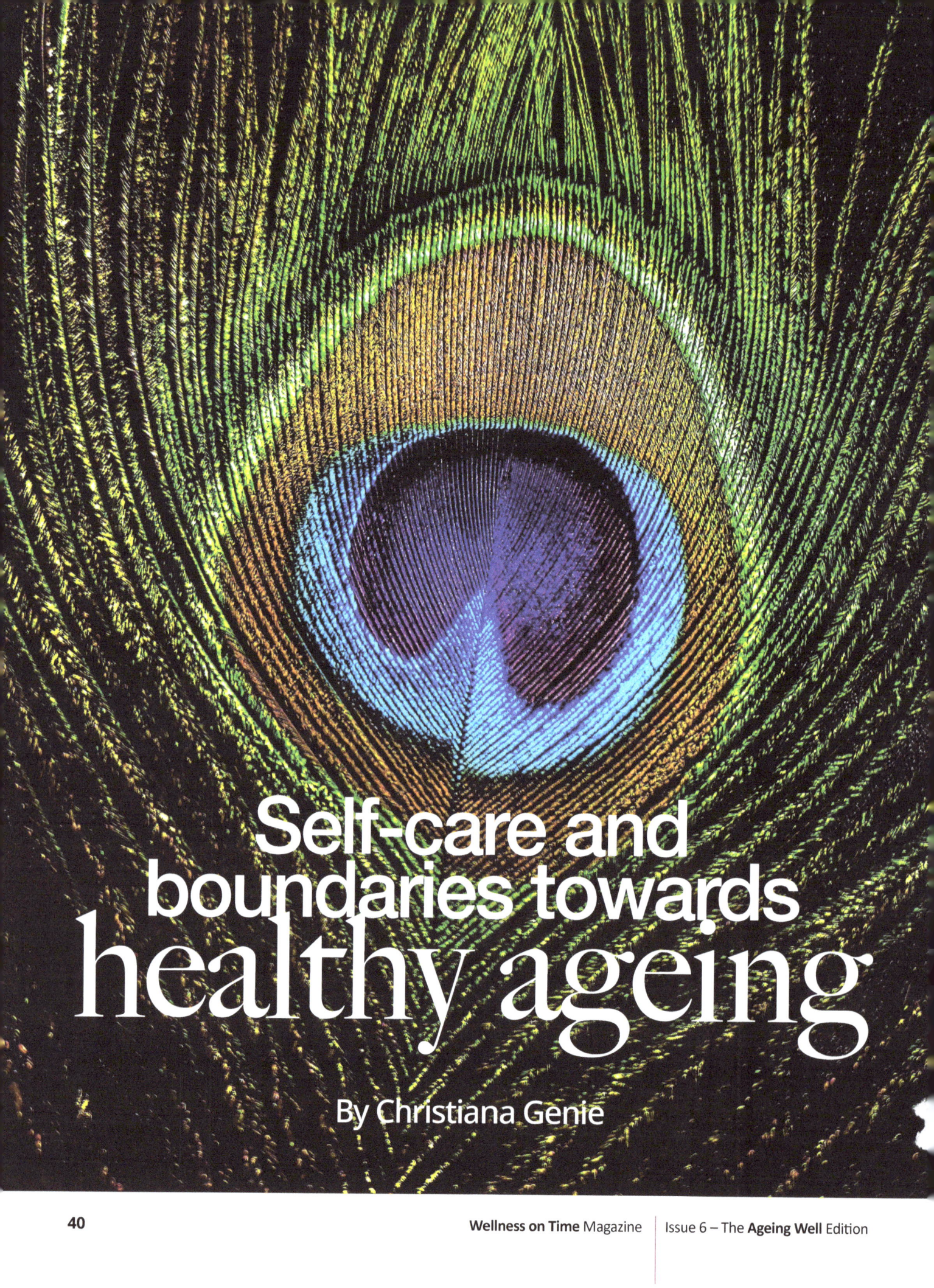

Self-care and boundaries towards healthy ageing

By Christiana Genie

Life had become a whirlwind, and before I knew it, I was on the verge of turning 40, facing the undeniable reality that I had navigated through half of my life. Yet many of the dreams and aspirations I once held seemed to remain unfulfilled. I found myself stuck in a dead marriage with two toddlers, a scenario where my soul was screaming for change, while my logical mind attempted to convince me that I was foolish to even consider such a drastic shift.

Eventually, the strain of suppressing my true desires took a toll. My body began to manifest the stress I was under, with severe vertigo being a clear message that something had to give. That was when I made one of the most difficult decisions of my life – I chose to end my marriage. In doing so, I stumbled upon a profound realisation – the importance of setting boundaries.

> That was when I made one of the most difficult decisions of my life – I chose to end my marriage. In doing so, I stumbled upon a profound realisation – the importance of setting boundaries.

The power of boundaries

Boundaries, with those around us and within ourselves, are vital to our well-being and essential for healthy ageing. For me, the process of setting boundaries began with the courage to stand up for my values, even when it meant disappointing those around me. One of the hardest truths I had to face was that the pain of others, particularly when it stemmed from my actions or decisions, was not mine to carry.

> One of the hardest truths I had to face was that the pain of others, particularly when it stemmed from my actions or decisions, was not mine to carry.

It was then that I began to see how I had been compromising my most cherished value – freedom. Throughout my life, I had always championed the freedom of others, whether that was through supporting human rights, animal welfare, or environmental causes. Yet I had neglected my own freedom, keeping myself trapped in a relationship that no longer served me, striving to be the perfect woman, mother, and professional, while ignoring my own needs.

Steps to healthy boundaries

Emerging from this experience, I've identified three essential steps to ensure that you set healthy boundaries, which in turn will support your well-being as you age:

1. Be clear on your values: understanding what is truly important to you is the foundation for setting firm boundaries. If you don't have a clear sense of your values, you will find it challenging to stand your ground when those boundaries are tested. Take time to reflect on your core beliefs and what truly matters in your life.

2. Speak your truth: it's crucial to express your needs and boundaries, regardless of how others might react. People are resilient and can handle disappointment. Remember, everyone is responsible for their own emotions, and failing to meet someone else's expectations is not your burden to bear. By being honest and direct, you honour yourself and those around you.

3. Accept negative emotions: setting boundaries can be accompanied by difficult emotions such as guilt, sadness, fear, failure, or anger. These feelings are a natural part of the process and should be acknowledged, not suppressed. Allow yourself to feel these emotions, recognise their presence in your body, and breathe through them. They are temporary visitors on your journey to a more fulfilled and balanced life.

> Allow yourself to feel these emotions, recognise their presence in your body, and breathe through them. They are temporary visitors on your journey to a more fulfilled and balanced life.

Embrace your humanity

It's important to remember that we are here on Earth to fully experience our humanness. Adapting to everyone else's requirements may seem noble, but it often comes at the cost of your health, particularly your immune system, and overall mental and physical well-being.

Setting boundaries is the secret ingredient to happiness and longevity. By establishing clear limits, you conserve your energy for personal growth and keep your cup full, enabling you to give to those you love from a place of abundance rather than depletion.

Healthy ageing isn't just about our physical health – it's also about our emotional and psychological well-being. By being true to yourself, setting boundaries that protect your values, and embracing the emotional journey that comes with it, you lay the foundation for a life that is not only longer, but richer and more fulfilling.

Christiana Genie is a Parenting and Life Skills expert.

Cortisol
The double-edged sword

By Cheri Shandra

Cortisol, or the 'stress hormone', is produced in our adrenal glands, the organ sitting comfortably above the kidneys. The adrenal glands receive signals from the hypothalamus and pituitary glands in the brain, which regulate the production of cortisol.

Cortisol is responsible for stress response. It also plays a massive role in maintaining our body's balance in various ways, such as:

> **Blood sugar:** working closely with insulin to maintain blood sugar levels, it converts protein into glucose
> **Inflammation:** works as a natural anti-inflammatory drug
> **Metabolism:** regulates how our body uses fats, proteins, and carbohydrates for energy
> **Immune system:** cortisol can boost the immune system by limiting inflammation
> **Sleep-wake cycle:** cortisol is naturally lower in the evening, making it easier to relax, while higher in the morning, aiding in energy.

Much like a home alarm system ready to alert owners to any intrusion, cortisol patiently awaits the brain's signal for alarm in the adrenal glands, allowing the hormone to release in the bloodstream and get to work.

Although we understand the importance of cortisol, we must be clear on what can occur when it floods the body and causes detrimental results. Released throughout the day, cortisol is higher in the morning and lower in the evening, yet fluctuating in small amounts as needed. When we perceive a person or situation as a threat, we release more significant amounts of cortisol as our body's primal response to remain alert and energised. This occurs after adrenaline (also known as epinephrine) is produced and released, which is a hormone and neurotransmitter responsible for our fight-or-flight response.

So, what happens when we remain in a consistent state of stress? Over-production of cortisol caused by prolonged and persistent stressful events can have detrimental effects on the functioning of our adrenal glands. Some of the physiological effects of prolonged cortisol release include:

> **Weight gain:** high cortisol levels cause stubborn weight, especially around the abdomen and face
> **High blood pressure:** contributes to hypertension
> **Skin issues:** rashes, acne, discoloration, and prolonged healing
> **Irregularity of menses:** delayed, missed, or heavy menstrual cycle flow
> **Fatigue:** feeling extreme bouts of exhaustion
> **Intestinal problems:** irritable bowel syndrome or episodes of constipation, diarrhoea, or bloating
> **Mood disturbance:** excessive cortisol results in anxiety and depression, linked to Cushing's Syndrome, an endocrine disorder linked with a variety of psychiatric and neurocognitive disorders
> **Low libido:** little to no desire for physical intimacy
> **Sleep disturbances:** instead of lessening in the evening under regular release, excessive cortisol causes higher levels later at night

> **Musculoskeletal tension:** the activation of the sympathetic nervous system during high-stress levels causes tension headaches, aching joints, and poor recovery from exercise.

The effect of prolonged high cortisol levels is becoming more widely accepted as a severe implication for one's health. Holistic health has long seen the correlation with ailments and the implication of one's environmental and emotional situations, seeing how it dramatically impacts the physiological responses of an individual. Today, we see that illnesses otherwise overlooked with a blanket diagnosis of chronic fatigue or chronic diseases are more commonly attributed to the extreme effects caused by a surge of cortisol due to stressful and traumatic events.

In my personal experience, I found myself losing a sense of who I once was. I could barely move without feeling the pang and prodding of irritable sensations throughout my body. I suffered from physical pain, hair loss, skin irritations, headaches, weight gain, irritability, and more.

I decided I needed to regulate my body holistically. I could no longer tolerate the way I felt. The answers I was receiving about my health left me more confused and stuck. I decided to research and explore how to heal, and I have also helped others do the same. Here are some things you can do right now to aid in your wellness:

> **Exercise:** 20 minutes daily can help reduce stress and induce productive sleep
> **Limit caffeine:** caffeine can increase cortisol levels
> **Mindful practices:** yoga, meditation, and somatic healing can all aid in lowering stress
> **Hobbies:** doing what you love can release endorphins and serotonin, the relaxing and happy hormones.
> **Go outside:** being in nature has many benefits, including promoting better mood, easier breathing, vitamin D, and improved focus
> **Supplements:** Ashwagandha, omega-3, magnesium, and vitamin C are some supplements that help your body adapt to stress by lowering cortisol. Always consult a medical professional before use
> **Nutrition:** foods rich in magnesium, fermented foods, dark chocolate, avocado, spinach, and more can help lower cortisol and maintain mental well-being. Pro tip: Serotonin, the 'happy hormone', is mainly made in the gut (about 95%!), so what you eat significantly affects your feelings.

So, even though cortisol is multifunctional in our body's ability to operate correctly, we must remain vigilant to keep regulated and stay proactive in our overall peace. Although not always possible to achieve, you deserve peace and serenity – especially knowing that this double-edged sword of cortisol can cause deep wounds in our overall wellness when not tended to.

Cheri Shandra is a board-certified Holistic Nutritionist, internationally accredited Trauma Recovery Practitioner, Founder of The Shandra Company and Creator of the Tangled in Toxic podcast.

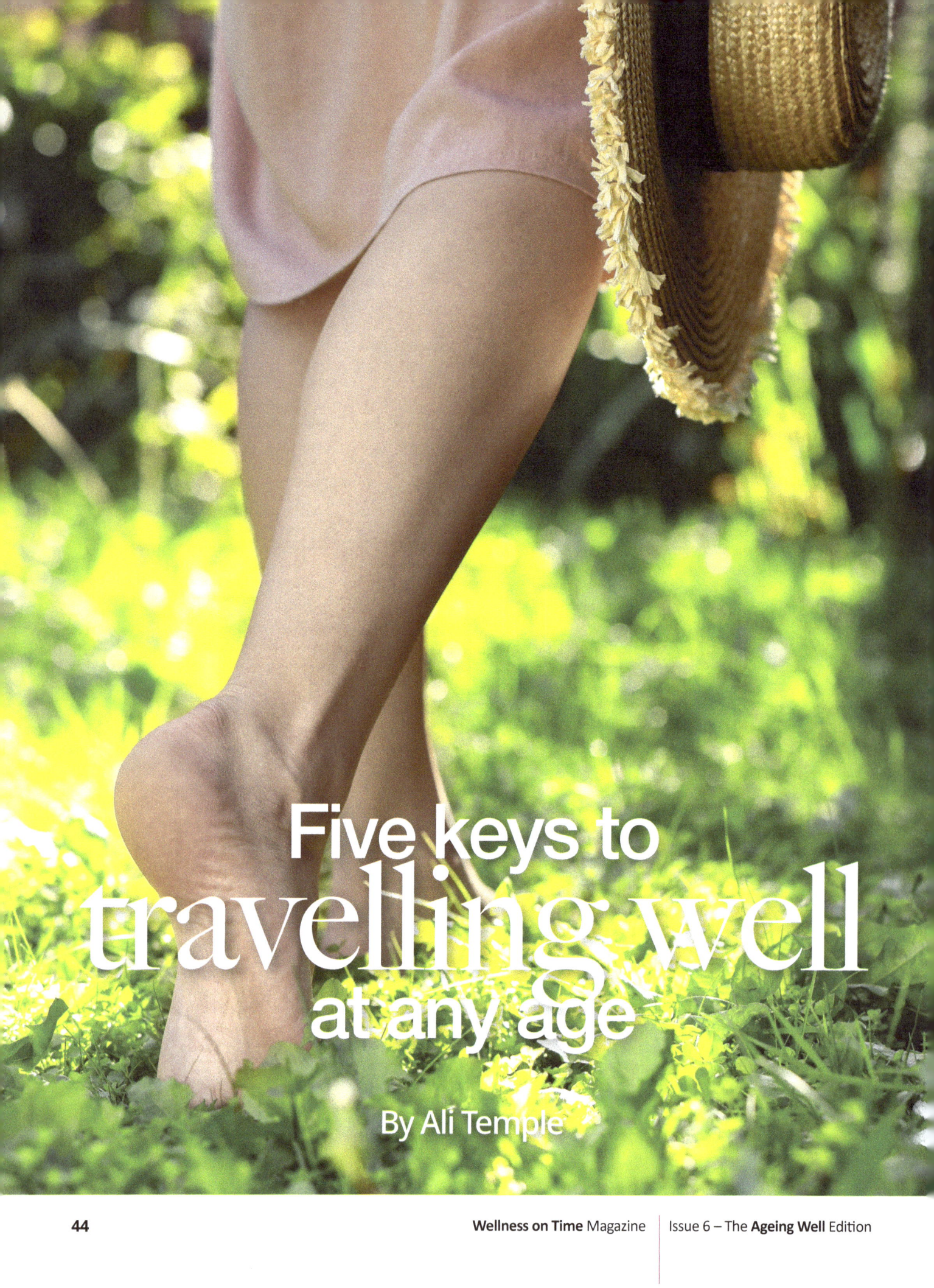

Five keys to
travelling well
at any age

By Ali Temple

As an almost 40-year-old female entrepreneur, I have spent the last four years travelling full-time, living out of a suitcase, and running my remote retreat and mentoring business. It sounds dreamy, doesn't it? But without a steady home base, and constantly moving to a new place every week or two, I found myself completely burned out. My health was suffering, and I knew I needed to make some changes.

So, I made a big decision – I moved to Bali. I thought that slowing down in this beautiful, serene environment would be just what I needed to get my health back on track. But life had other plans. Shortly after arriving, I contracted Dengue fever – a harsh wake-up call that sidelined me for three months. During that time, I realised just how out of balance I had become. My immune system was shot, and my nervous system was frayed. It wasn't until I chose to take my power back, focusing on rebalancing my life, that I began to truly heal.

As I approach my 40th birthday, I'm more committed than ever to sharing what I've learned along this journey. I'm passionate about empowering other women to live their travel dreams without compromising their health. So, here are my top five tips for staying well during travel at any age.

1. Embrace 'slow travel'

The biggest lesson I've learned is the importance of slowing down. When you're constantly on the move, your body and mind don't have time to adjust, which can very quickly lead to burnout. Slow travel isn't just about spending more time in each place, it's about allowing yourself the space to truly experience and enjoy your surroundings. By staying in one place for a month or more, you can find a routine, connect with the local culture, cook your own high-quality meals, and give your body the rest it needs to stay healthy.

> The biggest lesson I've learned is the importance of slowing down. When you're constantly on the move, your body and mind don't have time to adjust, which can very quickly lead to burnout.

2. Start your day with a grounding practice

One of the most stabilising habits I've developed is a consistent morning grounding practice. I start my day with Qi Gong, breathwork and if possible, stepping onto the grass outside my villa, and grounding with some deep breaths. Whether it's meditation, journaling, or simply enjoying a quiet cup of tea (device-free), starting the day with intention helps to centre your mind and body. This practice becomes even more important when you're travelling, as it provides a sense of stability and routine, no matter where you are in the world. I've found that taking just 15–20 minutes each morning to breathe deeply and set my intentions for the day can make all the difference.

3. Pack your comforts

When you're travelling, it's easy to feel ungrounded and disconnected. One way to combat this is by packing a few of your favourite comforts. When I started this location independent journey, I only had a backpack. I've since upgraded my packing several times and can honestly say I take no shame in living out of one full-sized suitcase plus one carry-on. When considering your 'comfort essentials', these might include essential oils, a cozy blanket, your oldest sweater, or extra packs of your favourite tea. For me, it's my pillow (yes, I'm the woman who travels with her own pillow!), and a small travel-sized diffuser that fills my space with the familiar scents of lavender and eucalyptus. Having these comforting items with me helps to create a sense of home, no matter where I am.

4. Stay connected to your community

Travel can be isolating, especially if you're constantly on the move. That's why it's crucial to stay connected to your community, whether it's friends and family back home or new connections you make on the road. In Bali, I've joined local gyms and yoga studios, which has helped me feel more supported and connected. Whether through virtual groups, video calls, or in-person meetups, maintaining these connections can provide emotional support and keep your spirits high.

5. Prioritise daily movement

Daily movement is key to staying well during travel. Whether it's a morning walk, joining a tennis club, or jumping into a pilates class, keeping your body active helps to reduce stress, boost your immune system, and improve your overall mood. I've made it a priority to move every day – sometimes it's as simple as a walk on the beach or rolling out my yoga mat at the villa (I've been teaching yoga for a decade and practicing for two). It doesn't have to be intense – a gentle movement practice is often enough to help keep your body and mind balanced.

Travelling is one of life's greatest joys, but it's easy to lose sight of your well-being when you're constantly on the go. By embracing slow travel, grounding yourself with a morning practice, bringing along your comforts, staying connected, and prioritising daily movement, you can enjoy the adventure without sacrificing your health. After all, the journey is as much about maintaining your well-being as it is about exploring new places. So go ahead, chase those travel dreams, and remember to take care of yourself along the way.

Travel well!

Ali Temple is the CEO of Ali Temple Yoga and Mentoring Inc., and Founder of the Traveling Wellnesspreneur Podcast.

From pain to power
New habits for enhanced quality of life

By Cécile Baumann-Arnold

Can you remember ever having back pain as a child? Yes, of course, many of us have suffered from stomachaches or toothaches, but overall, our bodies felt relatively free. There were hardly any chronic complaints or discomfort. However, this state often changes gradually and imperceptibly, influenced by performance pressure, the demands of time, hours of being sedentary, and the pressures of expectations.

It often starts with a slight discomfort and can escalate to chronic pain and restricted movement. I experienced this myself. By the age of 17, I was already dealing with chronic neck pain, a constant companion that not only brought discomfort but also extreme fatigue and an ongoing sense of unease that weighed heavily on my mood. Within just a few years, the life that once felt so carefree and joyful transformed into a burdensome struggle for survival.

How could this happen? Was there a way out? By the time I turned 25, having tired of my suffering and exhausted conventional therapies, I was ready for a profound change. That's when I discovered the Alexander Technique, which provided me with the answers to the 'How?' and 'What?' behind my situation.

Our bodies are designed with a fundamental structure that we instinctively use in our daily lives. However, throughout my education and even during my dance training, I seldom learned how to use this design in a health-promoting manner that could sustain vitality and energy over time. It often seems as if our bodies should operate seamlessly, without the need for special attention or consciousness.

As we instinctively imitate and adapt to our surroundings, many of us have developed a habit of leaning forward with our gaze toward screens, meetings, or exercise. This unconscious response causes our heads – each weighing about 4–5kg – to be pulled forward. The spine and trunk are designed to optimally support the head as long as the connection between the two remains intact. However, when the head shifts forward, movement muscles are activated to maintain this disadvantageous position. These muscles are not intended for this holding task, because their function is to enable movement.

Taking on this support function is akin to mistreating our own bodies. It leads to poor posture, and the pain that develops over time is communicated back to our brains. Yet do we understand what our bodies are trying to tell us? Do we know what changes we need to make?

While the Internet offers a plethora of information and exercises for neck pain, many of these remedies are often short-lived or only effective for as long as we actively practice them. To address the root cause of pain, the deeper knowledge needed is often lacking.

This is especially relevant as we think about ageing. The habits we cultivate in our youth and adulthood significantly influence how we age. Poor postural habits, lack of movement, and high stress levels can lead to early onset of chronic pain and mobility issues, all of which can severely impact our quality of life as we grow older. Conversely, adopting healthier habits, such as those promoted by the Alexander Technique, can enhance our mobility, reduce pain, and ultimately contribute to a more graceful ageing process.

Let's examine the factors that contribute to these pains:

> performance and time pressure
> extended periods of immobility while sitting or standing
> a tendency to focus our gaze toward goals (screens, smartphones, conversation partners)
> unconscious use of our biomechanical design.

The holistic approach lies in how we handle pressure, question our immobile postures while sitting and standing, and rethink our responses to stimuli (screens, etc.). It is essential to cultivate a greater awareness of our personal design.

Here are some simple steps you can take to feel better. Let go of what bothers you, reduce pressure, keep your eyes relaxed, and allow your head to move back over your spine, supported by your trunk. Release tension and discomfort, and permit movement while sitting and standing. Return to yourself and consciously observe your reactions to pressure and other stimuli. How could you respond differently? How can you ensure that you engage with your body according to its design, with mindfulness and kindness?

> How could you respond differently? How can you ensure that you engage with your body according to its design, with mindfulness and kindness?

The following mental instructions, often used in the Alexander Technique, can help you establish new health-promoting habits:

1. Can I take my time, notice my body, and remain mindful while engaging in this activity?
2. Am I allowing my body to be mobile and vibrant? Is my breath flowing freely?
3. Where am I unconsciously restricting my mobility? Approach this with curiosity and explore how your body functions. Numerous online resources can illustrate the anatomical workings of the body. Observe how your body naturally imitates these movements and strive to gain personal movement experiences. If your body resists certain movements, honour that reaction and don't force anything. Just being aware that these movements are possible can inspire your body to explore them mindfully and safely.

I hope this article inspires you to consciously observe your body during your activities, release tension, and develop new responses to stimuli. Embrace the journey of self-discovery and empowerment. Much success on your path to a healthier and more fulfilling life!

Cécile Baumann-Arnold is a Federally licensed Complementary Therapist and Member of the Swiss Association of the Alexander Technique.

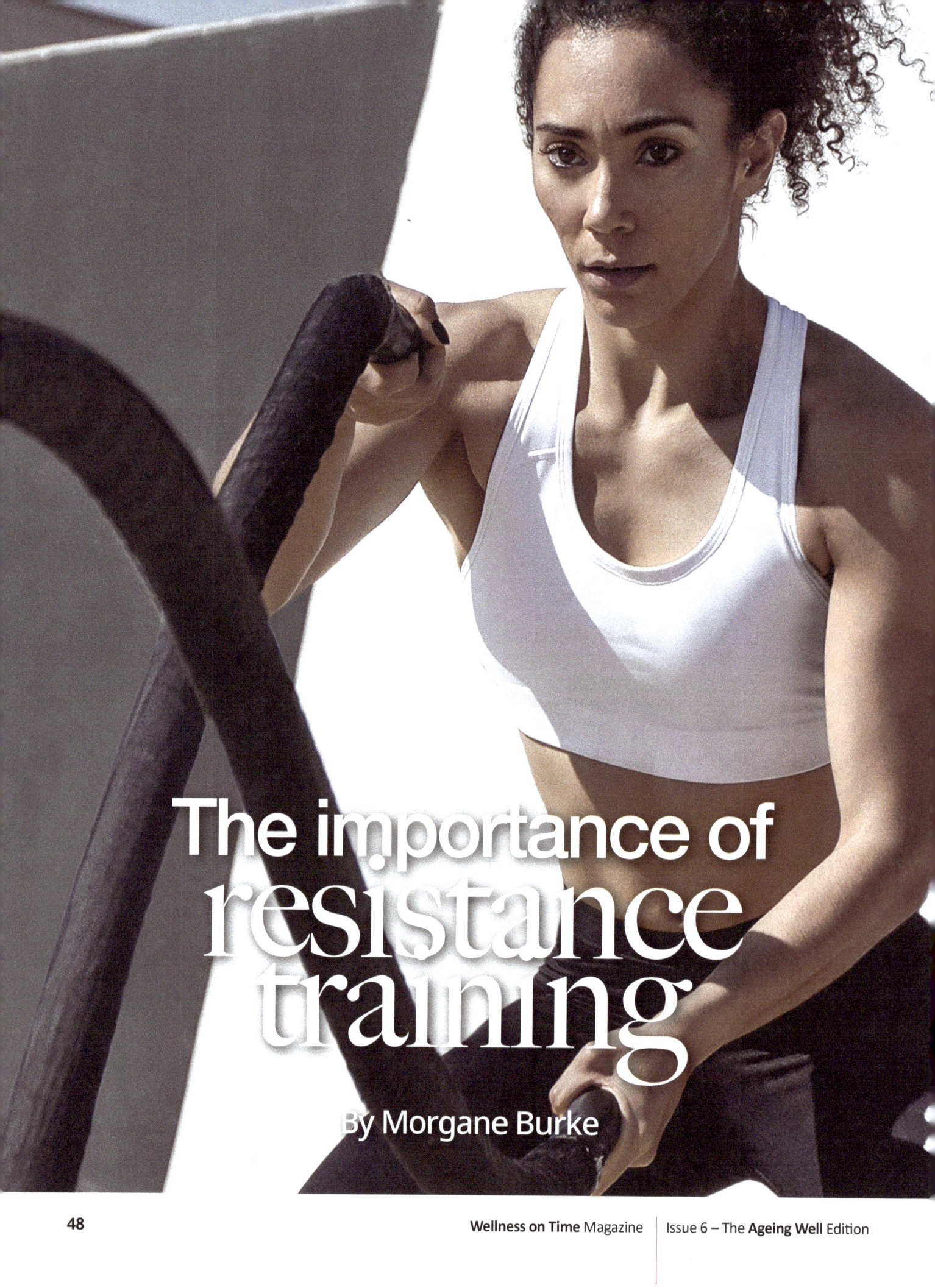

The importance of resistance training

By Morgane Burke

As a certified personal trainer and nutrition specialist who has been pretty active on social media, I am, for sure, the recipient of whatever algorithms are currently trending in the industry. I also have a front row seat for any type of speculation about what's the most efficient method to lose weight, tone up, increase energy levels, or tackle perimenopausal symptoms.

While most content seems to be encouraging and motivating, I also find this constant outpouring of information incredibly confusing for someone who is just starting on a wellness journey. 'Lift heavy and ditch cardio!', 'Run three miles a day!', 'Prioritise low impact exercises!', and/or 'Count macros and weigh your food!'

What's the right combo and what should be given the most focus? Well, if you ask me, it depends on (among other things) your goals, your history with training, your age, and your current health status. However, resistance training, in most cases, is non-negotiable.

Resistance training doesn't necessarily mean training to or close to muscle failure every single time, hitting scary gym machines, or only focusing on iron pieces of equipment. Sure, this is also part of it but a resistance band or even your own body weight can also work wonders!

> Resistance training doesn't necessarily mean training to or close to muscle failure every single time, hitting scary gym machines, or only focusing on iron pieces of equipment.

Why is resistance training so important?

What if I told you that a consistent resistance training routine will create the gap between a 60-year-old individual who experiences a common fall that only requires some icing, a few rest days, and maybe some anti-inflammatory medications in order to get back to their normal activity level, and a 60-year-old individual who experiences the same fall leading to a hospital stay, full or partial immobilisation, tremendous loss of muscle mass resulting in permanent handicap, and potential premature death.

Establishing a consistent resistance training routine is a crucial factor when it comes to longevity. Recent research has shown that metabolism does not necessarily slow down with age but is predicted by the amount of muscle mass. Starting around age 30, muscle mass naturally declines 3%–8% per decade. So, what do you think happens if we don't engage in consistent resistance training? Not only do we lose strength, but we also become more insulin resistant, fatigued, gain weight, and observe a drastic decrease of energy level and metabolic function, which combined may lead to a rapid acceleration of the ageing process.

I have been working with women of all age groups and have been witnessing the struggles that my perimenopausal clients in particular have been experiencing trying to come out of a sedentary lifestyle. They are hit with several symptoms including, but not limited to, drastic increase of visceral fat, fatigue, constant inflammation, impossible weight loss, and cravings. These symptoms are mainly due to a change in hormones (predominantly estrogen) that tends to control fat storage locations in the body.

Resistance training helps minimise or, in some cases, get rid of those symptoms by increasing metabolic activity and size of muscle fibres, as well as helping prevent osteopenia and osteoporosis. It also improves quality of sleep, which we know is absolutely essential for the regulation of appetite hormones.

Engaging in physical activity and particularly resistance training as early on as possible is key to ageing gracefully, making this dreaded stage of life much smoother for women.

> Engaging in physical activity and particularly resistance training as early on as possible is key to ageing gracefully …

I love cardio training and enjoy it two to three times a week. Cardiovascular health is very important as well, but I realise that as I am getting older, I will need to slowly shift the ratio in favour of resistance training. Practicing what we truly enjoy is so important, so if running long distances fills your cup, by any means, enjoy it and don't stop. After all, mental health has a significant key role in the ageing process, and movement is medicine.

Morgane Burke is a certified personal trainer and nutrition coach, Founder of Morgane Burke Fitness and Creator of Body Transformation Accelerator – Your 90 Day Roadmap to Looking and Feeling Your Best.

The key to living our dream life is following our joy.

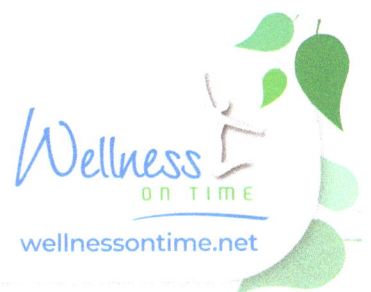

Wellness
ON TIME
wellnessontime.net

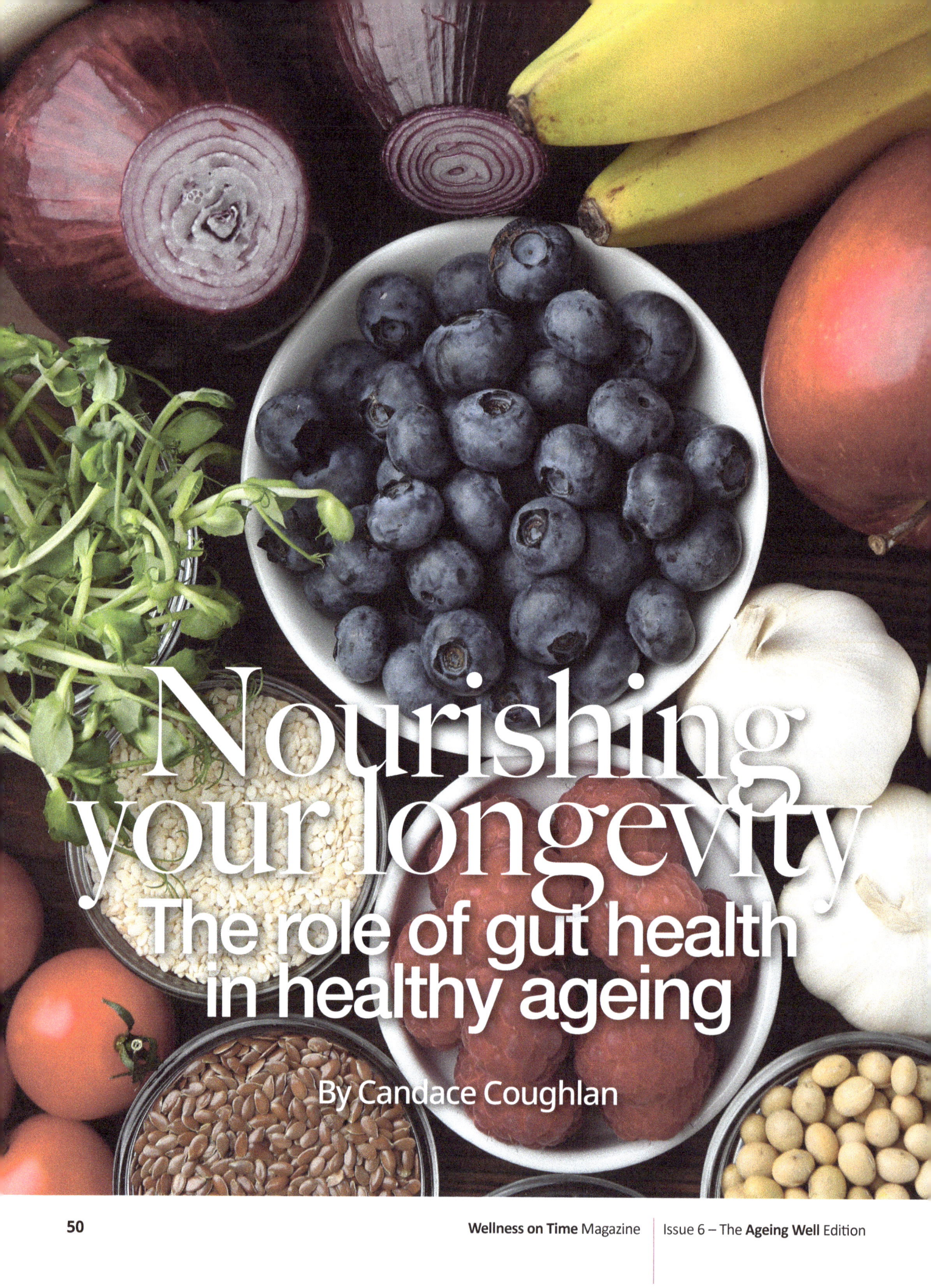

Nourishing your longevity

The role of gut health in healthy ageing

By Candace Coughlan

The journey to healthy ageing begins in a surprising place – your gut. The trillions of microorganisms that reside in your digestive system, collectively known as the microbiome, play a crucial role in your overall health. Emerging research shows that a balanced microbiome can be a key factor in promoting longevity and healthy ageing, helping to stave off age-related diseases and maintain vitality as you grow older.

Your microbiome is a bustling ecosystem that influences nearly every aspect of your health – from digestion to immune function and mental well-being. As you age, the diversity and balance of this microbial community tends to decline, which can lead to increased inflammation and a weakened immune response. This imbalance, known as dysbiosis, has been linked to various age-related conditions, including cardiovascular disease, diabetes, and cognitive decline.

Research has shown that maintaining a healthy microbiome can help mitigate these risks. A diverse and well-balanced microbiome supports the body's natural defences, reducing inflammation and bolstering immune function. Moreover, certain strains of beneficial bacteria have been associated with improved cognitive function and a lower risk of neurodegenerative diseases. Keeping your 'gut flora' in check is not just about digestion, it's about protecting your entire body as you age.

One of the most effective ways to support your microbiome is through your diet. The foods you eat directly impact the composition of your gut bacteria, making dietary choices a powerful tool for promoting longevity. Beyond the well-known benefits of a balanced diet, emerging evidence suggests that a diet rich in diverse, plant-based foods can create an environment where beneficial bacteria thrive, further enhancing your health as you age. Diets high in unhealthy fats and refined sugars have been shown to disrupt gut flora, emphasising the importance of mindful eating to sustain a healthy microbiome.

Fibre is essential for a healthy microbiome because it serves as food for beneficial bacteria. Consuming a diet rich in fruits, vegetables, whole grains, and legumes helps nurture a diverse microbiome. These foods provide prebiotics – non-digestible fibres that feed the good bacteria in your gut, encouraging their growth and activity. Regular intake of a variety of fibres can also help prevent constipation (a common issue as we age), by promoting regular bowel movements.

Incorporating fermented foods into your diet introduces beneficial bacteria, known as probiotics, directly into your gut. Foods like yoghurt, kefir, sauerkraut, kimchi, and miso are rich in these live cultures. Regular consumption of these foods can help maintain a balanced microbiome, reduce inflammation, and even improve digestion and nutrient absorption.

While probiotics are live bacteria that add to the population of good bacteria in your gut, prebiotics are the food that these bacteria need to thrive. Foods like garlic, onions, leeks, and bananas are excellent sources of prebiotics. Together, prebiotics and probiotics form a dynamic duo that supports gut health and overall health as you age.

Together, prebiotics and probiotics form a dynamic duo that supports gut health and overall health as you age.

Maintaining a healthy microbiome doesn't require a complete dietary overhaul. Small, consistent changes can make a big difference. Start by incorporating more fibre-rich foods into your meals, such as adding a handful of leafy greens to your lunch or opting for whole-grain bread. Fermented foods can also be easily added to your diet. Try starting your day with a probiotic-rich yoghurt or adding a spoonful of sauerkraut to your dinner.

Staying hydrated is another simple yet effective way to support gut health. Water aids digestion and helps keep the mucosal lining of the intestines healthy, providing a good environment for beneficial bacteria to thrive. Additionally, minimising the intake of processed foods and sugars can prevent the growth of harmful bacteria that contribute to dysbiosis. Incorporating herbal teas, which often contain gut-friendly ingredients like ginger and peppermint, can also support digestion and overall gut health.

For those interested in taking an active role in their gut health, home fermentation projects can be fun and rewarding. Fermenting your own vegetables, for instance, allows you to create custom probiotic-rich foods tailored to your taste and nutritional needs. Engaging in these projects can also provide a sense of accomplishment and a deeper connection to your food, further enhancing your commitment to a healthy lifestyle. The simple act of creating your own fermented foods can deepen your understanding of the importance of gut health in overall well-being.

The connection between a healthy microbiome and longevity is becoming increasingly clear. By making gut health a priority, you can take proactive steps towards ageing gracefully and maintaining vitality throughout your life. Whether it's adding more fibre to your diet, enjoying the benefits of fermented foods, or simply staying hydrated, small, consistent changes can have a profound impact on your overall health.

So, start today. Support your microbiome, and in doing so, support your health for a long, vibrant life.

Candace Coughlan is a gut-focused Culinary and Holistic Nutritional Practitioner, certified Integrative Nutrition Health Coach and Nutrition Educator, and Founder of Wild Health Hub.

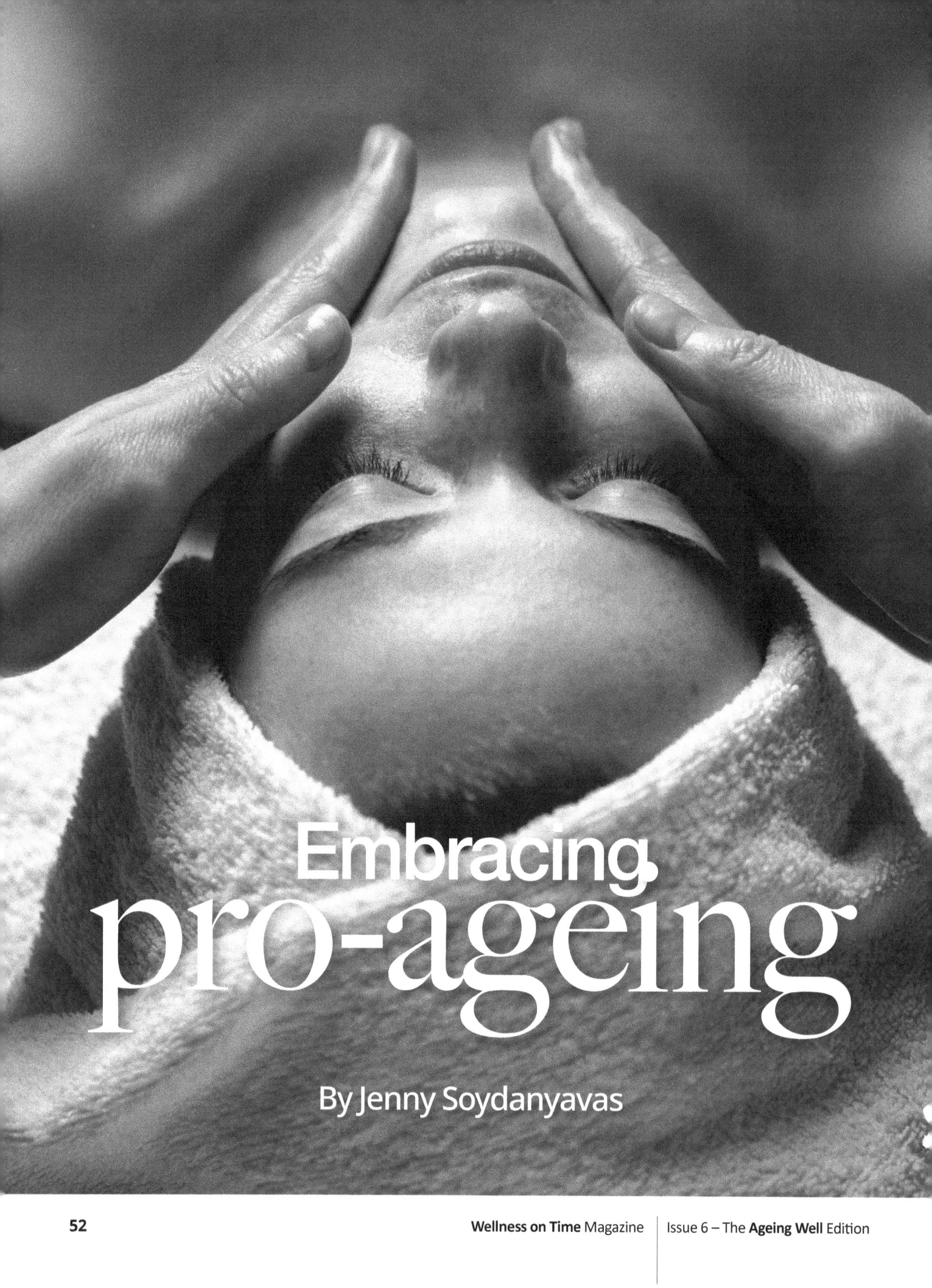

Embracing
pro-ageing

By Jenny Soydanyavas

Ageing is a privilege that we take for granted. Comments such as 'You look younger than your age' seem like compliments and enforce the idea that the younger you look, the better. We spend so much time and energy covering our grey hair, trying to smooth the wrinkles, and simply appearing younger. The mindset we want to celebrate is that older age is something to be celebrated and respected, and something full of wisdom and learning.

I want to share how embracing a pro-ageing mindset and adopting simple, yet powerful skincare rituals can help you feel confident in your skin. As I heard someone say recently, 'Beauty is a feeling, not a thing we look at'.

Embracing pro-ageing: a mindset shift

The term 'anti-ageing' is everywhere, promising us the secret to stopping time. But what if, instead of resisting the natural ageing process, we embraced it? Pro-ageing is about shifting the narrative to one that acknowledges the beauty and wisdom that come with age. It's about understanding that ageing isn't something to fight against, but something to live with gracefully and confidently.

By adopting a pro-ageing mindset, you're not giving up on looking and feeling your best. Instead, you're aligning yourself with realistic and empowering goals. The focus moves from unattainable perfection to nurturing your skin and overall well-being. When we stop resisting the natural changes in our bodies and start supporting them, we begin to cultivate a deeper sense of self-love and confidence.

Holistic skincare rituals: beauty is a feeling

One of the keys to supporting your skin as it ages is taking a holistic approach. This means going beyond the products you use and incorporating rituals that nurture your skin and your spirit. Techniques like facial massage and Gua Sha are gaining popularity, and for good reason. These practices don't just enhance the appearance of your skin, they promote relaxation and help you reconnect with your body.

Face massage, for example, stimulates circulation and helps relieve tension in the facial muscles, encouraging lymphatic drainage and promoting a healthy, radiant complexion. Studies show that just a few minutes a day of gentle massaging can soften fine lines, enhance skin tone, and improve your mood.

Gua Sha, an ancient Chinese healing technique, involves gently scraping the skin with a smooth tool to promote blood flow and ease tension. It's been shown to boost circulation, reduce puffiness, and improve skin elasticity. The result? Your skin looks more radiant and feels more vibrant.

These rituals are more than just skincare techniques – they are moments of self-care that allow you to connect with yourself on a deeper level and remind you to slow down and appreciate the beauty in the present moment.

Less is more for mature skin

As we age, our skin often becomes more sensitive, making it essential to simplify our skincare routines. While it may be tempting to reach for a shelf full of products, a minimal approach can often be far more effective for mature skin. This 'less-is-more' philosophy allows your skin to breathe and function naturally, while also minimising the risk of irritation.

As we age, the skin's ability to repair and protect itself slows down, so maintaining a healthy skin barrier becomes even more crucial.

A simple routine with a few high-quality, targeted products can deliver better results than overwhelming your skin with too many ingredients. I always recommend a gentle, oil-based cleanser, a hydrating and balancing beauty essence, and face oil.

High-performance ingredients: nature's allies

When choosing products for your pro-ageing skincare routine, focus on high-performance ingredients that work with, not against, your skin's natural processes. Many mature women find that their skin becomes drier and thinner with age, making hydration and skin-plumping ingredients essential.

One powerhouse ingredient to look out for is hyaluronic acid (a naturally occurring molecule) known for its ability to retain moisture, keeping your skin hydrated and plump. Included in your skincare products, it's perfect for reducing the appearance of fine lines and adding a youthful glow to the skin.

Another key ingredient is niacinamide, also known as vitamin B3. It's a multi-tasker that helps improve skin elasticity, enhances barrier function, and evens out skin tone. It can also reduce redness and blotchiness, making it ideal for sensitive, ageing skin.

Lastly, never underestimate the importance of antioxidants. I love antioxidant-rich Arctic berries in my skincare as they protect your skin from environmental stressors, such as pollution and UV rays while brightening and evening out skin tone. By using products rich in antioxidants, you help defend your skin against damage, keeping it looking vibrant and healthy.

Ageing is inevitable, but how we approach it can make all the difference. When we adopt a pro-ageing mindset, embrace holistic skincare rituals, and focus on minimalism and simply feel better, you can support your skin's natural functions and feel confident in your beauty at any age.

Jenny Soydanyavas is the Founder of Jenny Nordic Skincare, a Gua Sha Facialist, and Educator.

Empowering confidence

How permanent cosmetics transform the lives of older clients

By Tara Rebel

As the beauty industry evolves, one niche that has gained significant traction is permanent cosmetics. This field, also known as micropigmentation or permanent makeup, involves the application of pigments to the skin to enhance facial features. While it caters to a diverse clientele, one demographic that particularly benefits from these services is older adults. For many in this age group, permanent cosmetics studios offer more than just aesthetic enhancements – they provide a means to restore confidence and self-esteem.

My name is Tara, and I am the owner of Rebel Aesthetic Academy in Marlton, NJ. I am an American Academy of Micropigmentation certified expert in permanent cosmetics and scalp micropigmentation (SMP), and a platinum level American Academy of Micropigmentation (AAM) trainer/instructor of permanent makeup.

I discovered my niche in the beauty industry very early in life by being exposed to it through my family. After obtaining an Associate Degree in Education and a Bachelor Degree in Psychology, I decided I wanted to pursue my interest in the world of aesthetics. Realising my heart was also in the beauty industry, I decided to open my own business. As a perfectionist by nature, I have a keen eye for design with a passion for enhancing facial features using the latest techniques, the highest quality tools in the industry, and a custom design for each client and their specific goals. I have helped thousands of clients achieve their desired natural looking results, and I truly understand the power of looking and feeling great, 24/7.

The appeal of permanent cosmetics for older clients

Ageing is a natural process that brings about various changes in the skin, hair, and overall appearance. Thinning eyebrows, fading lip color, and less defined facial features are common concerns among older adults. These changes can significantly impact self-esteem, leading to a desire for solutions that help maintain a youthful and vibrant appearance. Permanent cosmetics studios address these concerns through personalised treatments that enhance natural beauty.

Eyebrow restoration: eyebrows play a crucial role in framing the face and conveying expressions. However, with age, eyebrows can become sparse or disappear completely. Techniques like microblading and powder brows have revolutionised eyebrow restoration. By implanting pigments into the skin, these methods create the appearance of fuller, natural-looking eyebrows. For older clients, this can make a dramatic difference, rejuvenating their facial appearance and boosting their confidence.

Lip color enhancement: as we age, lips can lose their natural color and definition. Lip blush and lip liner treatments are popular among older clients seeking to restore the youthful hue and shape of their lips. These procedures involve depositing pigments into the lips to create a subtle, long-lasting tint. The result is a natural looking enhancement that negates the need for daily application of lipstick or lip liner.

Eyeliner and lash enhancements: the delicate skin around the eyes is often one of the first areas to show signs of ageing. Permanent eyeliner and lash enhancement treatments help define the eyes, making them appear more awake and youthful. These procedures are particularly beneficial for older clients with vision issues or unsteady hands, as they eliminate the need for daily makeup application.

The emotional and psychological benefits

Beyond the physical transformations, permanent cosmetics studios offer significant emotional and psychological benefits for older clients. As individuals age, they may experience feelings of invisibility or a decline in self-worth. The ability to enhance one's appearance through permanent cosmetics can be incredibly empowering – fostering a renewed sense of confidence and self-assurance.

Restoring independence: for many older adults, applying makeup can become challenging due to physical limitations such as arthritis or tremors. Permanent cosmetics provide a long-lasting solution that reduces the need for daily maintenance. This not only saves time, but also restores a sense of independence, allowing clients to feel more self-reliant in their beauty routines.

Enhancing social engagement: feeling good about one's appearance can positively impact social interactions. Older clients who feel confident in their appearance are more likely to engage in social activities, fostering connections and reducing feelings of isolation. The boost in self-esteem from permanent cosmetics can encourage older adults to more actively participate in their communities and social circles.

The expertise and care of permanent cosmetics studios

Safety and precision: safety is paramount in permanent cosmetics. Reputable studios adhere to stringent hygiene standards and use high-quality pigments and tools to ensure the best outcomes. Practitioners undergo extensive training to master the techniques required for precise and natural-looking results. This level of professionalism is crucial in instilling trust and confidence in older clients.

Personalised care: each client's journey with permanent cosmetics is unique. Practitioners need to take time to understand their client's goals and tailor treatments to suit their needs. Whether it's creating subtle enhancements or more dramatic changes, the focus is always on achieving a look that complements the client's natural beauty and aligns with their desires.

Through specialised treatments and compassionate care, permanent cosmetics studios address the aesthetic concerns associated with ageing, providing a boost in confidence and self-esteem. The transformative power of permanent cosmetics goes beyond physical appearance, enriching the lives of older adults by restoring their sense of independence and enhancing their social engagement. As this industry continues to grow, it holds the promise of empowering more individuals to embrace their beauty at any age.

Tara Rebel is the Owner and Founder of Rebel Aesthetic Academy, a certified provider and trainer in permanent cosmetics and scalp micropigmentation.

The Lion King. Rated G. 89 minutes. Directed by Roger Allers and Rob Minkoff. Screenplay by Irene Mecchi, Jonathan Roberts and Linda Woolverton. Original songs by Elton John and Tim Rice.

Having stormed the box office when it was first released in 1994 (it remains the highest-grossing hand-drawn animation film ever made), this year celebrates the 30th anniversary of Disney's *The Lion King* – a flawless, enchanting rites of passage story that captivated, and continues to captivate, generations of filmgoers.

With the birth of his cub Simba (Jonathan Taylor Thomas), Mufasa (the late James Earl Jones) must ensure that his evil brother Scar (a perfectly sinister Jeremy Irons) understands that Simba must eventually assume his rightful place as the leader of the pride. Scar immediately joins forces with his henchmen – hyenas Shenzi (the brilliant Whoopi Goldberg) and Banzai (Cheech Marin) – to re-determine the course of the young cub's destiny.

> 'Everything you see exists together in a delicate balance. While others search for what they can take, a true king searches for what he can give.' — Mufasa

Certainly one of Disney's darkest affairs (with the death of Mufasa giving even the death of Bambi's mother a run for its money), *The Lion King* kicks into hyperdrive once the, now exiled, adult Simba (Matthew Broderick) meets the flatulent warthog Pumbaa (Ernie Sabella) and his theatrical companion Timon the meerkat (Nathan Lane). Timon and Pumbaa's impromptu burlesque to distract the enemy hyenas ('Are ya achin'/for some bacon?') is still a sensational example of Disney's determination to entertain their adult fans as much as the younger ones.

Hans Zimmer's Academy Award®-winning score is still as close as it is possible to be to the perfect accompaniment to all the colour and movement, while Elton John and Tim Rice's songs each serve the story beautifully – but none more so than the spectacular *The Circle of Life* sequence

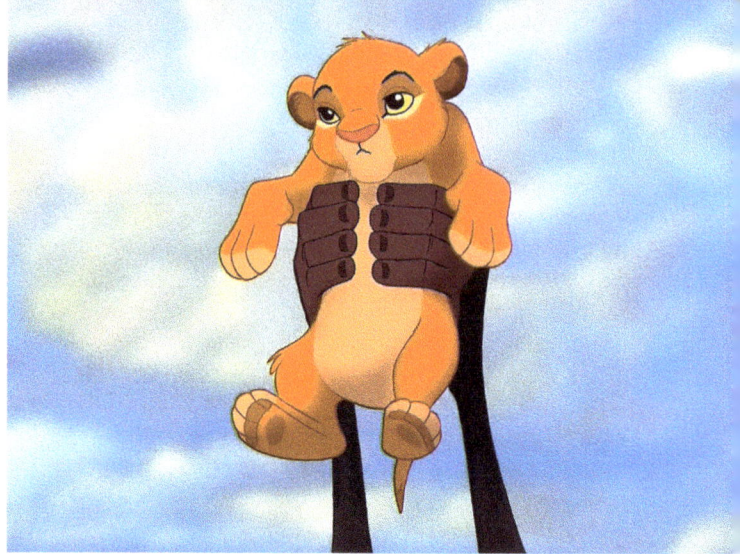

© Walt Disney Studios Motion Pictures

that remains not only one of this film's most memorable, but one of the finest opening sequences of any animated film ever made.

The stage adaptation by director Julie Taymor was an instant and spectacular success. *The Lion King* opened on Broadway at the New Amsterdam Theater on 15 October 1997 and went on to become Broadway's third longest-running show (after *The Phantom of the Opera* and *Chicago*) and the highest grossing Broadway production of all time, having grossed more than $1.9 billion. London's West End production, now in its 24th year, remains the West End's best-selling musical. Since its Broadway opening, *The Lion King* has played to an estimated audience of more than 110 million people worldwide.

The Lion King is streaming on Disney+. The stage version is currently playing on Broadway at The Minskoff Theatre, NY; the Lyceum Theatre, in London's West End; with productions also being staged in Toronto, Spain, France, Germany, Japan, Brazil, and on tour throughout North America. The origin story *Mufasa: The Lion King* is scheduled to be released in the US by Walt Disney Studios Motion Pictures on 20 December 2024.

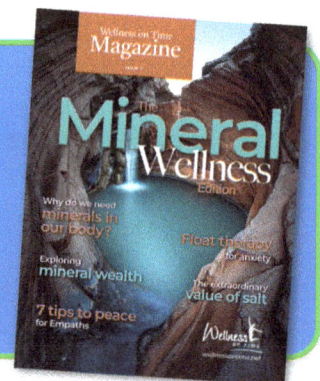

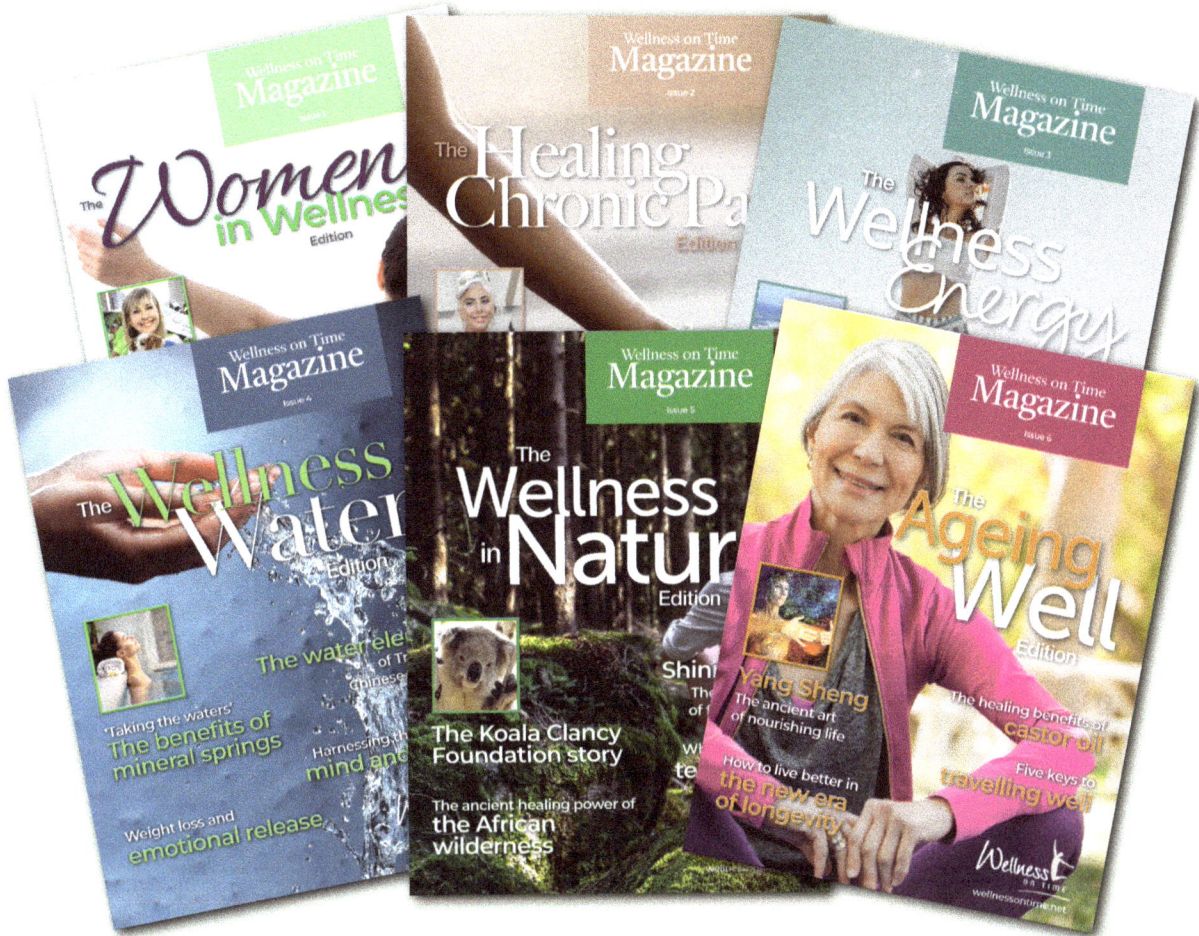

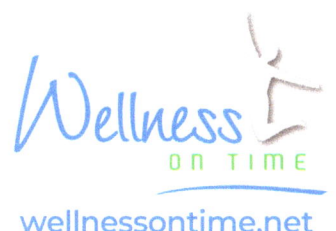

Is it time to change your thinking about how you exercise?

'Investing in your own health and wellness may turn out to be more valuable than investing in your retirement fund.'

Health, once it is gone, is very difficult to get back. Taking steps now to make positive changes to your lifestyle will most likely pay you dividends later.

Myth 1: No pain, no gain

The more that you enjoy it, the more likely you are to do it. Life should be fun, and exercise should be fun! In fact, studies show that at an excessive level, exercise can be detrimental to recovery for those under constant stress, which in our busy world is most of us! Gentle body movement, including breathing exercises, can be more beneficial than vigorous exercise – so do more of what makes you happy!

> Gentle body movement ... can be more beneficial than vigorous exercise – so do more of what makes you happy!

Myth 2: You need to do a 30-minute block otherwise there is no point

This is just not true, because doing something is better than doing nothing at all. What this 'advice' has done is suggest that when people look at the time they have available to exercise and realise they don't have 30 minutes to spare, they choose to do nothing rather than something. Even a 5-minute activity is better than no activity at all.

We've started you off by listing some activities on the notepad that involve moving your body to bring you joy. You can add some of your favourite exercise activities or make make notes about any observations that inspire you.

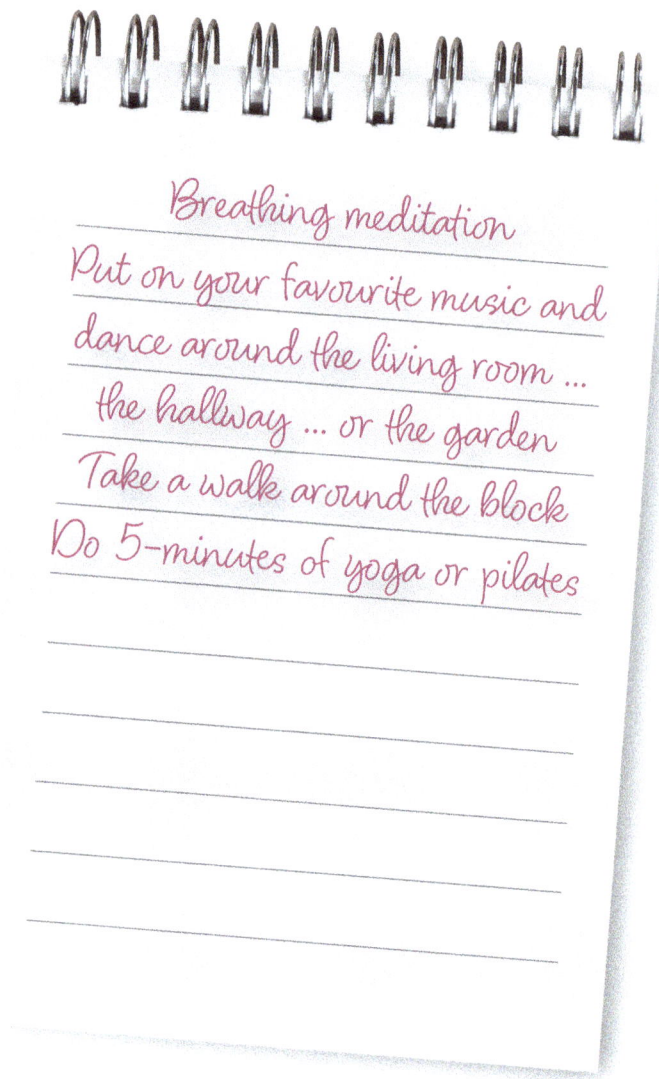

Breathing meditation
Put on your favourite music and dance around the living room ...
the hallway ... or the garden
Take a walk around the block
Do 5-minutes of yoga or pilates

Change happens through movement and movement heals.

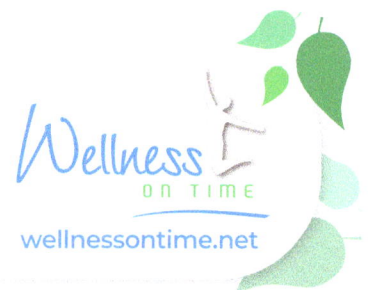

Wellness
ON TIME
wellnessontime.net

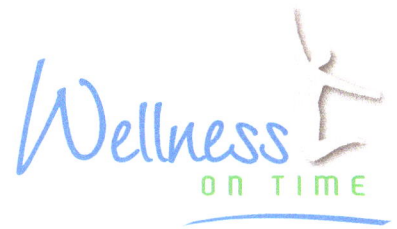